INFORMATION SICK

INFORMATION SICK

How Journalism's Decline and Misinformation's Rise Are Harming Our Health— and What We Can Do About It

JOANNE KENEN
LYMARI MORALES
JOSHUA M. SHARFSTEIN

JOHNS HOPKINS UNIVERSITY PRESS | *Baltimore*

© 2025 Johns Hopkins University Press
All rights reserved. Published 2025
Printed in the United States of America on acid-free paper
9 8 7 6 5 4 3 2 1

Johns Hopkins University Press
2715 North Charles Street
Baltimore, Maryland 21218
www.press.jhu.edu

Library of Congress Cataloging-in-Publication Data is available.

ISBN 978-1-4214-5312-5 (paperback)
ISBN 978-1-4214-5313-2 (ebook)

A catalog record for this book is available from the British Library.

Special discounts are available for bulk purchases of this book. For more information, please contact Special Sales at specialsales@jh.edu.

EU GPSR Authorized Representative
LOGOS EUROPE, 9 rue Nicolas Poussin, 17000, La Rochelle, France
E-mail: Contact@logoseurope.eu

CONTENTS

Preface vii

Acknowledgments ix

    Introduction: Information Sick   1
1. The Collapse of Local News   9
2. The Fracturing of National News   41
3. The Flood of Misinformation   67
4. The Innovators   96
5. By and For: The Rise of Community Journalism   117
6. The Playbook   137
7. Protecting Yourself—and Others   156

Notes   163

Index   193

PREFACE

By definition, it's tough to write a book about news, especially when the 24/7 news cycle seems to unfold in milliseconds rather than hours or days. Much has happened in the world of health since we started this book; more will happen by the time people read it. But our goal was never to recapitulate the headlines. It was—and is—to help explain how changes in the American media, and the ever-changing mix of information sources, are affecting the health and well-being of millions of Americans.

But of course, the headlines keep coming. As we write these words in May 2025, the United States is facing the largest measles outbreak in decades. One reason for the infection's rapid spread is the sidelining of traditional information sources, with a smorgasbord of opinions and "alternative facts" taking their place. What's happening with measles reflects what's been happening with many other health issues—from COVID to cancer, from diet to diabetes. The challenge runs much deeper than a single health issue, a single political figure, a single agency, or even a single election.

For decades, mainstream news outlets dominated national coverage, and local journalists in newspapers around the country sought stories of both interest and importance to relay to their audiences. Public health agencies worked with journalists to explain outbreaks of infectious disease and to offer the latest health guidance to the public. Communications was a tool for translating scientific advancements and essential information to hundreds, thousands, or even millions of people at a time—and for saving lives.

But that world is gone. Local newspapers are fewer and smaller, and people are more likely to get news from social media sites that are a mash-up of information, misinformation, and gossip. Public health officials have to contend with misunderstanding and mistrust proliferating across platforms. Deep partisan schisms have made it increasingly difficult to find even small patches of agreement.

Communications have shifted from a way for people to learn together about health to a highly individualized experience without a safety net. And for millions of Americans, the information they do receive is making it more difficult to protect themselves and their families from serious illness, injury, and even death.

We call this condition "information sick." This book focuses on describing this malady, tracing its origins, and mapping potential remedies. We hope it proves useful to all working to advance health and well-being.

ACKNOWLEDGMENTS

The authors gratefully acknowledge the Johns Hopkins Bloomberg School of Public Health for the opportunity to learn and teach about our changing information environment. We especially appreciate the consistent support and wise counsel of Dr. Keshia Pollack Porter, chair of the Department of Health Policy and Management, and Dr. Ellen J. MacKenzie, dean of the School.

Josh and Joanne thank the students and teaching assistants of the class that was the inspiration for this book. Teaching assistants Julie Ward, Kelsey Crowe, Odia Kane, and Ross Hatton had important insights across the subject matter covered in this book. They also thank the journalists, public health and misinformation experts who generously brought their wisdom (and warnings) to our classroom. Some of their voices you will hear directly in the book, but all of the guest speakers shared insights that were valuable to us and our students. They included Ricardo Alonso-Zaldivar, Drew Altman, Richard Besser, Helen Burstin, J Brian Charles, Caroline Chen, Rachel Chernaskey, Dave Chokshi, Meredith Cohn, Renée DiResta, Eric Eyre, Carrie Feibel, Sam Fromartz, Sam Fulwood, Hannah Furfaro, Rebekah Gee, Amy Goldstein, Luz Gray, Dianna Hunt, Nada Hassanein, John Hillkirk, Abby Johnston, Robert Lang, Shefali Luthra, Fairriona Magee, Graph Massara, Andrea McDaniels, Charles Ornstein, Alex Rabin, Elisabeth Rosenthal, David Rousseau, Margot Sanger-Katz, Beth Schwartzapfel, Tara Kirk Sell, Margo Snipe, Claire Wardle, Clinton Watts, Kytja Weir, Brandy Zadrozny, Alissa Zhu. In addition to the guest speakers, we also appreciate the journalists we interviewed for the book; you will meet them as you read.

Lymari thanks the hard-working and talented communications and marketing team at the Johns Hopkins Bloomberg School of Public Health, who have found success with creative and innovative approaches to public health communication. She is also grateful to the Bloomberg School students she has been fortunate enough to teach and engage with on these topics. She thanks her many teachers and colleagues throughout her career, and her family and friends who champion and support her.

Josh offers a special thanks to his wife Yngvild and his children Sam and Isa, who assure him that as soon as he learns about a new social media platform, it is no longer cool.

Joanne thanks her family, who agree with Josh's kids. Also the Commonwealth Fund and its former president David Blumenthal, which enabled her to come to Johns Hopkins, and the ABIM Foundation, which has included her in their forums on trust and communication in health, which has given her a framework for much of this work.

Finally, we acknowledge our fantastic research assistants, Julie Ward and John Poulos.

Introduction

Information Sick

In April 2022, National Public Radio (NPR) told the story of a mom named Stephanie and her two daughters, Laurie and Vikki.[1] Stephanie had been an attentive parent who took her daughters for regular doctor's visits and made sure they were fully vaccinated. Laurie and Vikki grew up healthy and eventually started families of their own. Just before the pandemic, however, Stephanie began to forward videos to Laurie and Vikki—strange videos. The topics included "JFK Jr. is still alive; reptilian aliens control the government." Then, after the pandemic began, the videos she sent claimed that the new coronavirus was a hoax.

According to NPR reporters Geoff Brumfiel and Meredith Rizzo, "When the COVID vaccines came along, Stephanie absolutely refused to get one because she falsely thought the shots contained tiny microchips. Moreover, she began avoiding her daughters, who had gotten vaccinated, because she believed false information that the vaccines were being used to somehow spread COVID."

When Stephanie became ill with COVID-19, she turned to unproven drugs promoted by the conspiracy videos she had been watching. After she was taken to the hospital, she refused treatments authorized by the US Food and Drug Administration. Her daughters watched helplessly as her condition turned from bad to worse.

"We all said goodbye and told her she was the best," Laurie said about her mom's passing. "I don't believe she was supposed to die. . . . I blame the misinformation."

Something is deeply amiss in America.

It's not just that more than one million Americans died from COVID-19, at a rate higher than all but a few countries in the world. Americans die from more preventable and treatable causes than the residents of all our peer nations. More than 100,000 Americans died in 2023 from drug overdose.[2] Suicide rates are rising.[3] Life expectancy has been stagnant since 2017 and fell dramatically during the pandemic.[4] Newborns in more than 35 nations now can expect to live longer than a baby born in the United States.[5]

Underlying these terrible headlines are shocking gaps in health. Native Americans and Alaska Natives, for example, have a life expectancy of about 65 years—more than 10 years shorter than the white population.[6] Black Americans die at a higher rate from heart disease;[7] Black Americans and Hispanic Americans are much more likely to die from diabetes.[8] Rural Americans kill themselves three times more often than their urban counterparts.[9]

In previous eras, science and policy drove vast improvements in health. After water quality experts proved that chlorination was safe, policymakers invested in water treatment plants. Once scientists invented a vaccine to prevent polio, parents lined their kids up for shots. As physician researchers discovered breakthrough treatments for both common and rare ailments, including cancer, legislators expanded access to medication coverage in the Medicare program and later health insurance through the Affordable Care Act.

Today, however, science has lost its luster. The percentage of Americans who say that science is a positive force in the world has dropped precipitously, as has the share who have confidence that scientists act in the public interest.[10]

Americans are actively turning their backs on life-saving interventions. Just about 38 percent of Americans in nursing homes—and only 15 percent of staff—were up to date as of January 2024 on COVID-19 vaccines as recommended by the Centers for Disease Control and Prevention.[11] More parents are refusing to vaccinate their children,[12] and some are even refusing vitamin K shots, which prevent hemorrhage in newborns soon after birth.[13] Some adults are turning their back on cancer chemotherapy to try widely touted but evidence-free alternatives.[14] Adolescents are self-diagnosing mental health conditions based on videos from influencers, leading to confusion and delays in treatment.[15] There is widespread misunderstanding about and discrimination against effective treatments for opioid addiction, preventing people from getting life-saving help.[16]

The Annenberg Public Policy Center at the University of Pennsylvania runs FactCheck.org, a service that debunks misleading information online. In early 2024, the website's posts included the following:[17]

- Blood donations from COVID-19 vaccine recipients are safe, contrary to online claims
- Comedian Amy Schumer has endometriosis, not a vaccine-related ailment
- Posts mislead about measles, MMR vaccine amid recent outbreaks
- Viral posts misuse rat study to make unfounded claims about COVID-19 and autism
- OJ Simpson Died from Cancer, Not COVID-19 Vaccine

In 2021, the single most popular Facebook post across the world, viewed billions of times, told the misleading story of a doctor who died after receiving the COVID-19 vaccine.[18] It is no surprise that from mid-2021 to mid-2023, trust in the medical system dropped sharply, from 44 to 34 percent, according to a Gallup poll.[19] Attacked, disbelieved, underfunded, and frustrated, doctors, nurses, and other health professionals are quitting their professions in droves.[20]

In 2023, *The Washington Post* investigated the decline in US life expectancy but found little interest among policymakers in taking on the challenge directly. With few exceptions, elected officials and appointed federal health officials alike described the problem as too difficult, too diffuse, too polarized, and too complicated to prioritize.[21] No doubt policymakers recognized the challenge of identifying, let alone advancing, a common health agenda.

Today, more knowledge is readily available than at any other time in human history. With just the tap of a finger, it is possible to access information about recent discoveries, advice from the world's leading experts, and millions of scientific papers. This democratization of information could have propelled America along the road to health.

Instead, the 21st century has proved hazardous to truth, with deadly consequences.

In short, America is information sick.

This book aims to explain this condition, its underlying causes, and its potential treatments. And that starts with the big picture: Health is not alone. What's happening to trust in public health, medicine, and science is happening to trust generally in institutions across society—falling "precipitously" over roughly five decades.[22] A Gallup poll on Americans' views of 16 institutions—from Congress to business to the media—found most had the confidence of half or less of the country. That poll found, too, that growing numbers of people perceived "made up news" as a big problem, and that it was undermining "our confidence in each other."[23]

Online debate, as internet expert Renée DiResta writes, had degenerated into a "new system of persuasion—influencers, algorithm, and crowds—[that] was radically transforming what we paid attention to, whom we trusted, and how we engaged with each other." A debate over facts has been displaced by what DiResta calls "a war of memes," with warriors ranging from Russian intelligence to anti-vax entrepreneurs. The casualties include health leaders and institutions.[24]

As trust plummets, facts themselves seem up for grabs. A Pew survey found that nearly three-quarters of Republicans and Democrats said that not only can they not agree on policy with those in the opposing party, they can't even agree on the facts.[25] And that was in 2019, before COVID-19, before the events of January 6, 2021, before all the rest of the political and societal disruption of the past few years.

In *The Anatomy of Deception: Conspiracy Theories, Distrust and Public Health in America*, Sara Gorman describes the interplay between threats to democracy and threats to public health. She writes, "During the

COVID-19 pandemic, trust declined not only in the arena of healthcare but also in political and governmental institutions as well. The failure of communication during a crisis, as witnessed especially during the early days of the COVID-19 pandemic, is really a symptom of an ailing democracy and not simply a matter of training public health professionals to communicate better."[26]

America's information sickness is a consequence of journalism's decline. Hundreds of local newspapers have closed, undermining community cohesion, civic participation, and community health. Online sites, from Facebook to Reddit to Nextdoor, may plug in a few of the gaps and create some cyber-niches that give a sense of community. But they tend to be more useful for finding a lost cat or recommending a plumber than they are for holding local government officials accountable or sharing consistently factual and trustworthy health news.

National media has shrunk, with only a handful of truly national papers remaining and the attention paid to policy, including health, receding. The three traditional television networks have survived, but their audience is now splintered by cable and online outlets that are often politicized. Many local television stations, newspapers, and radio stations are now owned by ideologically driven networks. Nationally, the popularity of the ideological pundit has led to a deep polarization of the airwaves. In more than a smattering of cases, local and national outlets, in a struggle to survive, have resorted to artificial-intelligence-generated news articles.

Coinciding with the crisis in journalism is the explosion of social media, which enables falsehoods to spread around the world and back instantaneously. The problem is deeper than a misleading tweet or Facebook post. Nation-states are deliberately spreading falsehoods for political gain. WhatsApp users spread lies on closed chat groups that link thousands of people across continents.[27]

The result is doubly dangerous to health—more bad information, less good information. More voices attacking science and public health; fewer able to distinguish between expertise and nonsense. More confusion, cynicism, and conflicts of interest; less clarity, optimism, and independence. All against a backdrop of declining trust and deepening social and political divides.

In addition to describing and analyzing this challenge, this book sets out solutions. Even at this challenging moment, it is possible to find glimpses of progress—starting with new information sources devoted to exploring health challenges and pointing the way to the solutions. These include nonprofit news sources like ProPublica, KFF Health News, The Trace, The Marshall Project, and the Food and Environment Reporting Network. They also include emerging media serving communities of color and other underserved groups, such as Capital B, the 19th, *The Nevada Independent en Español*, and many more. These organizations are fighting to overcome what Benjamin Toff and colleagues have called news avoidance, a phenomenon that keeps people from seeking critical information even when their lives may depend on it.[28]

There are also examples of universities and health centers stepping up to communicate essential information to the public, as well as new techniques for health care professionals and public health leaders to fight back against distortions and untruths. The old playbook of issuing a press release and calling a couple of reporters to make news is far past its expiration date. Surviving—and even thriving—requires an office of communications fluent in social media and ready to move quickly.

We wrote this book for everyone who is distressed about the unfortunate state of information and health in America—from public health commissioners to community clinicians to concerned citizens. Our goal is to explain what is happening in the world of journalism and social media, its profound consequences for health, and what can be done now to fight back.

Chapters 1–3 focus on three dimensions of the problem: the crisis in local news, the polarization of national news, and the explosion of misinformation on social media and beyond. These chapters explain how massive shifts in the economic and political landscape of US media now represent potent threats to health.

In chapter 1, we introduce Eric Eyre, a longtime reporter for a feisty newspaper in West Virginia who won a Pulitzer Prize for jaw-dropping reporting on the drug distributors dumping millions of opioid pills into the state. That paper has been sold: Eyre is no longer doing daily journalism. His story helps to understand the erosion of local news across the country, and how it is harming health.

In chapter 2, we introduce Ricardo Alonso-Zaldivar, a veteran reporter who spent most of his 43 years in the news business covering health, including for the Associated Press. Wire service reporters used to help set the agenda for the national news. But the national media too is now much more fragmented, politicized, and hyperfocused on electoral horse races. Social media, unvetted and often unreliable, competes for attention. Policy news, including health coverage, gets short shrift. So do the American people.

In chapter 3, we introduce Brandy Zadrozny, an NBC reporter whose beat is "disinformation." She spent a year searching for a nurse named Tiffany Dover, who had been hounded into hiding after conspiracy theorists insisted she had died from the COVID-19 vaccine. The chapter explores how misinformation and disinformation are spreading faster than they can be contained, and examines some of the emerging, but as yet insufficient, tools to try to combat them.

In chapters 4 and 5, we turn from harm to health—and focus on new and emerging trends in the media environment that are bringing high-quality information to the public, including to populations long overlooked. This is encouraging—but there is not yet enough of it to counter all the negative and damaging trends.

Chapter 4 examines a broad range of new publications that are focusing on health and public health topics, from violence to food to the environment. We introduce Alissa Zhu, a local reporter who left journalism for a public health degree, only to be pulled into the *Baltimore Banner*, a new nonprofit media venture in Baltimore. She was among the *Banner* reporters who took part in an award-winning reporting project on opioids with *The New York Times*.

Chapter 5 centers on new nonprofits that are giving voice to communities that have traditionally been underserved and unheard, and who are often targeted by misinformation, much of it health centered.

We introduce Dianna Hunt, a longtime journalist and Cherokee Nation descendant lured out of retirement by the opportunity to be senior editor of *Indian Country Today*, now a multimedia news platform known as ICT. She says she knows the publication is having an impact when readers spontaneously send contributions, some as low as five dollars.

Our final two chapters contain recommendations for rising to the challenge of information sickness. Chapter 6 offers guidance to public health agencies, universities, health care organizations and professionals, and policymakers—both for how to work with the media in today's world and for how to counter misinformation. And finally, in chapter 7, we end with a few tools and words of advice to the public on how to clean up the information environment, for the benefit of families, friends, and communities.

The late scholar and Senator Daniel Patrick Moynihan famously said, "Everyone is entitled to his own opinion, but not to his own facts." In the United States today, that is no longer the case. Stephanie, the conspiracy-minded mother of Vikki and Laurie, likely lost her life because she believed her own facts.

There is no reason to believe that being "information sick" in America is a self-limiting condition. It is unlikely to go away on its own. But neither is it untreatable. Learning what's happening and what can change is the place to start.

• CHAPTER 1

The Collapse of Local News

To understand the challenges facing local news, a good place to start is with Eric Eyre.

A longtime resident of West Virginia, Eyre wrote for the *Charleston Gazette-Mail*, a family-owned West Virginia newspaper, which traces its history back more than a century to a weekly established in 1873. Under the ownership of the Chilton family, from 1912 to 2018, the *Gazette-Mail* became a small paper with big journalistic ambitions, allowing reporters to pursue time-consuming projects of interest to their local community.

In 2007, Eyre was able to spend six months probing why West Virginians had such poor oral health and what could be done about it. He also wrote about meth labs, diabetes, and why his state consistently ranked so poorly in nearly every metric of health.

The newspaper wasn't just a chronicler of the state's daily events; it was a watchdog. It didn't just cover stories, it uncovered them. The scrappy *Gazette-Mail* had exposed corruption and greed and incompetence. No newspaper had reported on the coal industry more rigorously. The paper's Ken Ward Jr. was widely considered the nation's best coal reporter. His doggedness led to mine safety reforms and put corrupt coal barons in prison. The paper's tenacious reporting extended to state government, schools, local business, city hall, cops, and courts. It was an undeniable check on power.[1]

A decade later, Eyre helped uncover the breadth of the opioid crisis, including the role of "pill mills" and multinational drug distribution companies that sent literally millions of pills into small communities.

It was not easy going. The paper became embroiled in a series of court battles as it attempted to document and bring to light the actions of opioid distributors in West Virginia—and several of those battles were with the state itself, particularly its then–Attorney General Patrick Morrisey. Eyre reported on Morrisey's ties to the pharmacy industry and his wife's work as a lobbyist. In response, Morrisey didn't just demand records from the paper. He demanded voluminous, intrusive financial records, documents, and emails—and he wanted them fast. "The *Gazette-Mail*, one of West Virginia's most important institutions, was under siege," Eyre later wrote in his book *Death in Mud Lick*.[2] The paper eventually prevailed. Eyre's exposés on how the drug distributors had drowned West Virginia in opioids won the Pulitzer Prize for Investigative Reporting.

But even as the paper, the sole morning daily in the West Virginia state capital, was winning those accolades, the Chilton family could no longer hold on in a worsening economic climate. The paper had earned and held the community's trust for decades, but trust was hard to monetize. Advertising revenue was falling, as ads moved to the internet. Instead of paying for a subscription, people could find much of the content on free sites, notably Facebook. The *Gazette-Mail* filed for bankruptcy, and in March 2018 the Chilton family sold.[3]

The new owner was a regional chain that already owned several newspapers in the state. The chain transformed the economic model of the *Gazette-Mail*, drastically cutting costs. Resources dwindled; quality plummeted. As Eyre later told us, reporters started decamping, leaving town, and in some cases leaving journalism.[4]

The *Gazette-Mail*'s home page is now dominated by wire services stories; the local coverage has less depth and not much of an edge. There's a lot of sports news.

"It was a real roller coaster of a couple years," Eyre recalled. "We got the Pulitzer in April 2017. Eight months later, the *Charleston Gazette-Mail* . . . the paper that I worked at for 22 years, went bankrupt."[5]

Like many of its best reporters, Eyre quit, taking years of knowledge about West Virginia government, politics, and its struggles with health with him.

Patrick Morrisey was elected governor of West Virginia in November 2024.

The Vanishing Local Paper

In the late 20th century, not only did most communities in America still have a local paper, they had local papers, plural. Their reporters chronicled school board meetings, zoning decisions, health fairs, weddings, and obituaries. They kept an eye on local officials. Thanks to retail advertising, circulation revenue, and classifieds, they were also profitable.

Local media had deep connections to the people they served. Residents saw the reporters, editors, and even the publishers around town or knew them personally. People covering the community lived in or near the community; some had been born and raised there. This familiarity and commitment bred trust. Indeed, surveys by Gallup and the Knight Foundation have consistently found higher levels of trust in local than national news.[6]

But now, local news is dying. Print persisted after the "disruption" of radio, survived the arrival of television (although afternoon papers started folding as local evening news crept into their space), and even limped through the early years of the internet age. But small and midsize community newspapers have not survived the current amalgam of internet, smartphones and social media, and their cannibalization of advertising and classifieds revenue.

Local newspapers have been folding nearly every week, creating what are called news deserts. In fact, since 2005, the country has lost more than 1 in 3 of its newspapers; on average, about 2 papers have closed per week since 2005—nearly 2,900 papers, according to a 2023 research program on news deserts, now based at Northwestern University.[7]

Researchers at Northwestern identified 204 counties that were news deserts in 2023—and identified 228 more that were at "substantial risk" of becoming news deserts in the coming years. That means "no newspapers, local digital sites, public radio newsrooms or ethnic publications."[8] And despite some bright spots here and there, the overall trends in local news remains grim.

Despite innovation, partnerships, and nonprofit start-ups in some communities, many counties in poorer and more rural communities are truly in an information vacuum, some lacking high-speed broadband to connect them with other reliable news.[9] According to the Pew Research Center, 40,000 journalists—most of them local reporters—lost their jobs between 2008 and 2020. And the shrinkage continues.[10] Some little papers that are still publishing and purport to be local don't even have a staff beyond one reporter, or maybe a freelancer or two. Certainly they don't have a reporter doing deep dives into public health. Most of the content of these so-called ghost papers is produced elsewhere by a parent company and republished in these small local outlets purporting to cover their towns.[11]

As the famed investor Warren Buffett, who purchased some papers to make money (and not as part of his wide-ranging philanthropic ventures), said of local print newspapers as he dumped them, "It went from a monopoly to franchise, to competitive to . . . toast. . . . They're going to disappear."[12]

Weak or absent local news coverage has consequences. Stories that oversimplify or wrongly portray mental illness make it more difficult for compassionate policies to gain support. Those that stigmatize substance use reinforce ineffective approaches to policing and enforcement. Stories that confused the public about the Affordable Care Act made it more difficult to have reasonable conversations about its benefits and drawbacks.

The threat to quality local coverage was articulated at least as far back as 2009. In "The Reconstruction of American Journalism," an analysis of the news industry, then–*Washington Post* executive editor Leonard Downie Jr. and Columbia Journalism School professor Michael Schudson warned, "What is under threat is independent *reporting* that provides information, investigation, analysis, and community knowledge, particularly in the coverage of local affairs. Reporting the news means telling citizens what they would not otherwise know." Tim McGuire, a former editor of the Minneapolis *Star Tribune*, was quoted as saying in that report, "It's so simple it sounds stupid at first, but when you think about it, it is our fundamental advantage. . . . We've got to tell people stuff they don't know."[13]

When local journalism is not able to tell people what they don't know—and especially if they can't tell people what they may need to know—there are many consequences for health. The dearth of good local health reporting creates less awareness, less accuracy, more false equivalence, more distrust, and more confusion. It reduces accountability, of local government and local public health authorities. It also throws open the doors to more misinformation and disinformation—misleading individuals and families and disrupting care.

Take the example of Keith Smith, a 52-year-old engineer and married father of two who lived in York County, Pennsylvania. After contracting COVID-19 in November 2021, he became seriously ill and was admitted to the intensive care unit of a University of Pittsburgh health system hospital. His wife, Darla, began a frantic online search for a way to save his life. She found at least four newspapers that had reported favorably on how a few critically ill patients given the medication ivermectin had survived, including an 80-year-old woman in the Buffalo, New York, area.[14]

The problem was that ivermectin had never been demonstrated to be effective for COVID-19; studies would later show it is not effective.[15] But those upbeat reports prompted Darla Smith to sue to get her husband ivermectin.[16] She connected to an attorney who had received a lot of news coverage for ivermectin lawsuits, and the Front Line COVID-19

Critical Care Alliance, a group that was still promoting ivermectin. The court forced the hospital to allow an outside provider chosen by Smith to provide ivermectin. Soon after the second dose, however, Keith Smith died.[17]

As more papers close or scale back, among the job positions first to go are those dedicated to health reporting. Some papers don't even bother to cover health anymore, or only run wire service stories or free content from other medical sources—which, even if accurate, do not provide local connection and context. More reporters with health expertise end up leaving their jobs or being forced out. Eyre himself was forced off the health beat—and that was well before the paper was sold.

The closure of a local newspaper is not just an "Isn't it a pity?" moment, a whiff of nostalgia, a hurdle to finding the high school football scores or bulb-planting tips from the local garden club. It is far more damaging. As Margaret Sullivan documents in her book *Ghosting the News: Local Journalism and the Crisis of American Democracy*, the loss of quality local journalism hurts the health of communities in the broad sense. It leads to weakened community bonds, higher municipal spending, and decreased civic engagement, including lower voter turnout. Local officials have less accountability when there are no reporters to show up at local meetings, be it the city council, the county commissioners, or the school board.[18] And when local news dies, it throws the door open to misinformation and disinformation, some of it deeply injurious to health.

Trouble in the City

The little dailies and weeklies of small-town America aren't the only papers affected. Another tier of once influential newspapers, those from midsize and large cities, are also shadows of their former selves. These big-city papers were both local and in a sense national. They may not have been sold in newspaper boxes on street corners across the United States, but they had national aspirations and national influence.

This category includes papers like *The Baltimore Sun* and the *Chicago Tribune*. Or the *Miami Herald*, which was an international paper with a huge following in Latin America. These papers had bustling Washington bureaus and in some cases foreign correspondents. They informed their readers about their communities but also their country and their world.

Not anymore. There is perhaps no better example than the once venerable *Baltimore Sun*, which was on a path of excellence a few decades ago. It was a local paper but was also known for its national and international coverage, at one point in the 1980s having eight foreign bureaus. It now has none. It had a big health science and medicine team, partly because Baltimore itself was such a hub, home to both the authors' own Johns Hopkins University and the University of Maryland's health and medicine programs.

In the mid-2000s, for example, *The Baltimore Sun* identified challenges facing children with asthma, adults with HIV, and the environmental health of communities in South Baltimore. Each exposé created space for Baltimore's health department to announce new initiatives and policy changes. After the *Sun* reported and editorialized on a rise in the city's infant mortality rate, the attention generated momentum for a citywide effort to improve birth outcomes.[19] This effort, called B'more for Healthy Babies, has led to historic declines in the rate of infant mortality and in racial disparities in infant mortality.[20]

By this time, however, the paper was already enduring a series of sales and mergers and downsizings and reconfigurations. Then, in 2021, Alden Global Capital, a hedge fund that has come to symbolize a lot of what's befallen small and midsize papers, acquired it and the shrinkage continued. Less than three years later, in January 2024, Alden sold the *Sun* and several smaller Maryland newspapers to David Smith, chairman of the Sinclair network of conservative local television stations. It was a return to local ownership of the *Sun*—but Smith's initial meeting with the newsroom, including his conservative advocacy and his admission that he barely reads newspapers, did not raise expectations for improvement.[21]

Andrea McDaniels left the *Sun* after a 21-year career and is now the managing editor of *The Baltimore Banner*, a start-up nonprofit news outlet (discussed further in chapter 4). She had been a business reporter, a health and medicine reporter, and an editorial writer. When she started on the business desk in 2001, she was one of more than 20 reporters and editors. She was later one of about 10 health and medicine reporters. By the time she left, the *Sun* newsroom had fewer than 70 people total and the health team had shrunk from around 10 in the early 2000s to 1 or 2.[22]

"You can just imagine how the coverage changed. It just became harder to cover everything. I mean, we couldn't cover everything," McDaniels said. "The *Sun* had covered agencies and government and had great enterprise and great investigative pieces. As it shrunk, and got smaller and smaller, we became more of a reactive publication. We would cover city council meetings, we would react to police coverage, but we did less and less. Less enterprise. Less community reporting."[23]

Another example is the *Chicago Tribune*, which now is also a shadow of its legendary greatness. As McKay Coppins wrote in *The Atlantic* of his first visit to the Alden-acquired paper,

> After a long walk down a windowless hallway lined with cinder-block walls, I got in an elevator, which deposited me near a modest bank of desks near the printing press. The scene was somehow even grimmer than I'd imagined. Here was one of America's most storied newspapers—a publication that had endorsed Abraham Lincoln and scooped the Treaty of Versailles, that had toppled political bosses and tangled with crooked mayors and collected dozens of Pulitzer Prizes—reduced to a newsroom the size of a Chipotle.[24]

Former *Tribune* reporter Peter Kendall wrote a lot about health, science, and the environment for the paper before rising to become the editor of a large and ambitious health and science team and then managing editor. "The way history played out, my entrance into management exactly coincided with the beginning of the great contraction of newsrooms across the country," he remembered. "So when we had to decide between a health writer or a politics writer, that was often my agonizing call."[25]

Then what Kendall called the "Era of Evil Owners" began. He was sacked when the hedge fund took over. It was just after he had put on the front page the first few stories about a mysterious respiratory illness identified in China. Looking back on the *Tribune*'s glory days, he recalled that reporters and editors were initially thrilled by the internet, assuming strong legacy news outlets would be providing boatloads of profitable and fascinating content to all those web pages. Alas, he said, "the internet didn't need, or maybe even want, much of our content."[26]

Similar stories are playing out nationwide. Papers in cities as varied as Phoenix and Denver and Sacramento and New Orleans have scaled back, existing as skeletal versions of their more robust former selves. Once locally owned, many have now been acquired by chains, like the *Charleston Gazette-Mail*, or, like the *Sun*, by hedge funds or private equity companies.

Between 2002 and 2019, the share of papers owned by private equity firms had risen from 5 percent to 23 percent, including some in large markets, according to a 2022 working paper from the National Bureau of Economic Research.[27] Some of these new owners are trying to run decent news outlets, in difficult economic environments. Others have basically reduced newsrooms to the bare minimum, extracting profit and diminishing the value of the news. They have done more rounds of layoffs and reduced or eliminated print editions, going fully online.

According to the 2022 working paper, which is considered the first major study of private equity in journalism, the new ownership generally leads to a boost in digital circulation—and lower chances that the paper will close completely. But "the composition of news shifts away from local governance, the number of reporters and editors falls, and participation in local elections declines."[28] Instead of local news, the private equity firms rely more on national news stories—which can be printed in multiple newspapers at no extra cost. The hole in local news, however, is not plugged.²⁹

Consolidation of Local Radio and TV

As newspapers disappear or become shadows of their former selves, local radio and TV, in trouble themselves, have been unable to fill the gaps. Perhaps surprisingly, a lot of people still listen to radio, though not necessarily as their primary news source. A Pew study found that 82 percent of Americans aged 12 and up listened to radio in any given week in 2022, a drop from nearly 90 percent before the pandemic but still a big audience. Nearly half of adults get at least some of their news from radio, with the figures skewing toward people over age 50. But only one in five reported getting local news from radio, which is comparable to the numbers for the shrinking local newspapers.³⁰

And the radio they are listening to has changed.

The old "all news" local radio stations are largely gone; only about a score remain, mostly serving large cities, and even those outlets typically switch over to sports-dominated programming in the evening.

Baltimore still has several news and talk radio stations. The largest is WBAL, which brands itself NewsRadio. The station has news updates every half hour, 24/7, with several extended newscasts throughout the day. The day's programming also includes locally produced talk shows and live sports, including coverage of the Baltimore Orioles and Baltimore Ravens games. But WBAL too has undergone change. Robert Lang, who anchors or coanchors the noon and late afternoon broadcasts and still does a fair amount of enterprise and breaking news reporting, has seen those changes. He's been at WBAL since 2004, and spent nearly 20 years in smaller radio markets before that.

Lang's a local boy, Baltimore born. As a kid, he could see WBAL's radio transmitter towers from his backyard. He's old enough to remember rotary phones and landlines; in those days, if the wires weren't properly insulated, they could pick up WBAL and he could hear it on the phone, including Orioles baseball games. "I learned early on that broadcast journalism was what I wanted to do. And it was a goal of mine to work in Baltimore, and WBAL Radio has been committed for decades to covering local news and having its own radio news department," he told us. Until the early 1980s, Baltimore had four or five local radio stations, and the Federal Communications Commission required all stations to air a certain amount of news and public affairs programming. So even music stations had at least a few people who went out and gathered news, until the rule was eliminated as part of broader changes to electronic media industry regulation under the Reagan administration. As Lang explained, "The requirement for news was lifted. A lot of radio news teams and news departments disappeared."[31]

Lang's job, as he put it, is to "take very complicated issues, very complicated stories, and boil them down to a report that'll run 30 to 40 seconds on an hourly newscast." It is, he said, "a very simple presentation." Readers are listening to a live broadcast, often while they are driving or multitasking, one ear on traffic and weather reports. That doesn't mean there's never a longer, more detailed report, but it's not the rule, although WBAL did in-depth special reports, up to an hour long, on the coronavirus. Breaking news dominates, and radio reporters know how to jump onto the day's top stories—even if it means scrapping another piece they put a lot of time into. "If something major happens, you're interrupting programming and you're changing your rundown, your plan. You could have a beautiful, beautifully produced piece that doesn't make it on the air because of breaking news."[32]

But increasingly, both because Lang's an anchor and because the nature of newsgathering has changed, he's in the studio, rather than running around town or dashing off to Annapolis, the state capital. Sometimes, he said, that's frustrating. Nowadays, public proceedings are live streamed, so he can get the audio, say from a hearing in the state legislature, for his broadcast. But a live stream isn't the same thing as reporting in person. Lang's been around so long that he has good sourcing. But for newer reporters, it's harder to develop good source relationships—crucial to deeper, more contextual stories and for good watchdog reporting—with someone you've never met, if you are communicating by email or text. And even for Lang, live streaming and texting are not the same as being there. "What you miss are the people in the rooms. Their reactions. Seeing which lawmakers may be falling asleep," he said. Without being there, it's harder to know what's going on—and even harder to know what might happen next.[33]

WBAL is a throwback. The radio dial is increasingly dominated by highly political and polarized content. Rush Limbaugh pulled radio to the right starting in the 1980s, and his incessant pummeling of Bill Clinton's health care plan was among the reasons for the plan's collapse in 1994. Recently, the Salem Radio Network has been growing fast, serving up conservative and Christian-oriented news and talk shows.[34] Its daily hosts have included right-wing figures like Charlie Kirk and Sebastian Gorka. (Some of its lineup changed after the 2024 election and people shifted jobs.) Its shows have included AAR Daily Defense Hour; the initials stand for Armed American Radio. In contrast, an effort to build a liberal radio network, Air America, was short lived, ending in 2010.[35]

Meanwhile, local TV is facing its own challenges. Once upon a time, local television could unify a community. Actor Will Farrell and his castmates in the *Anchorman* movies may have famously parodied that—but the connections can be real and they can matter. As Wendy Rieger, a popular former TV reporter and anchor based in Washington, DC, put it upon her retirement, local TV is "a communal fire we gather around."[36]

But now local TV is undergoing its own transformation, partly because of legislative and regulatory changes to the communications field since the mid-1990s. A 2003 rules change from the Federal Communications Commission, for instance, let companies own more outlets. A follow-up in 2017 allowed a company to own both a radio and a newspaper in the same market. These changes facilitated big corporate rather than more local ownership, and large national companies bought up scores of local stations. This often meant more news segments, including health and medical news, were shared among multiple stations serving different communities. Even if accurate, these reports did not respond to local conditions or needs.

The poster child for the changes to local TV news is the Sinclair Broadcast Group, led by David Smith, who purchased *The Baltimore Sun* from its hedge fund owners. Since Sinclair's humble beginning as a radio training school in 1958 and its acquisition of its first TV station in 1960, it has become the largest owner of television stations in the United States. As of 2023, it owned or operated 185 stations in 86 markets. It gets about 80 million unique visitors a month, including for regional sports programming.[37]

Sinclair stations tout themselves as local news, but a substantial amount of content—often stories and commentaries with a right-leaning tilt—is reproduced essentially verbatim across the country.

Even in stations that haven't been swallowed up by the big chains or by those with a political tilt, TV journalists, like their print counterparts, are doing more with less. And the nature of the medium means they often don't have a whole lot of time to tell a complicated story.

"It's tougher. Newsrooms have fewer resources these days," said Angela Chen, a morning anchor at KESQ News Channel 3, which serves the Coachella Valley in California and which still has owners committed to covering their community. Sometimes, on her big medical enterprise projects, she actually can do a story that lasts seven minutes, maybe even seven and a half. That's a very long time for a local TV report. More typically stories are a minute or two. On a complicated topic, "it's pretty tough to explain, to do interviews, to get 'color,' and to do all of that within two minutes," she said.[38] With support from the University of Southern California Center for Health Journalism, she did an in-depth report on aging and family caregiving; earlier she did a big project on the Salton Sea, an environmental disaster with significant health implications for the region.

"Medical reporting—it's tough because you have to have a knowledge of medical systems and how they work. . . . When you get someone new into it, the reporting is not going to be in depth," Chen said. And the fact that the ranks of experienced reporters and editors, with institutional knowledge, is thinning out makes it harder for the less experienced reporters to learn. Of the veterans, she said, "They are retiring or they're going somewhere else and they are being bought out."[39] And many younger reporters—people who really wanted to be reporters—are so low paid that they are leaving the field.

Political scientists have found that as local stations get bought up, there's less local news coverage, less local political news coverage—and a lot more national news, mostly of politics.[40] Health coverage changes too.

In the early 2020s, a research collaborative on media and health messaging at the University of Minnesota, Wesleyan University, and Cornell University found that local television did a reasonably good job of covering obesity in ways that emphasized social, political, and food industry factors rather than just blaming individuals for gaining weight. Similarly, coverage of tobacco use began focusing more on the industry and social forces and less on the smoker.[41] But these nuanced approaches were not the rule. Local news, the researchers found, generally did not explain well how the Affordable Care Act could help people get covered, focusing instead on the political conflict. And that's becoming more of a trend in local TV health coverage in general. As the local news sector faces more competitive and economic pressure, reporting on health and medicine becomes more centered on conflict and sensationalism—and with fewer journalists on the health beat to provide health context. Boiling health news reports down to the length of a tweet on the station's feed might capture eyeballs "but may also produce health content that is more vulnerable to errors and omissions."[42]

The future looks even more grim. Cable retransmission fees have given local stations revenue, but with the shift toward streaming services, "cord-cutting," and an aging viewership, the economic future of local television, still a trusted source of news in much of the country, is deeply uncertain.

Slime Fills the Void

As quality local news reporting declines—whether in newspapers, on radio, or on TV—and eventually disappears, the information vacuum does not stay empty for long. However, much of what's now calling itself local news may be anything but. Indeed, some critics have labeled it "pink slime."

"Pink slime" is a term coined some years ago to describe meat filler added to ground beef. The phrase has been repurposed to describe hundreds of websites pretending to be sources of local news. They may have down-home and legitimate-sounding names like the *Eagle Times*, the *Glendale Sun*, even *Coachella Today*.[43] And they often perform well on Google searches, "appearing just below government pages, 'potentially adding to [their] credibility.'"[44] But they don't have real local reporters. The websites use the same articles from city to city, with some pseudo-local customization. Much of the content is bot-produced and then cloned to hundreds of "local" sites. Researchers at Columbia Journalism School's Tow Center for Digital Journalism and the Center for Media and Democracy at the Duke Sanford School have found that these sites are largely funded by a network of right-wing conservative donors and "dark money," which is hard to trace.[45] Follow-up research, published in 2024, found that "payments can be traced to organizations tied to conservative megadonors, including shipping magnate Richard Uihlein, billionaire tech investor Peter Thiel, and oil and gas billionaire Tim Dunn."[46]

Some online "news" sites have also been funded by groups promoting a liberal or progressive agenda that have not been transparent about the money or political connections.[47] In addition, there has been an increase in partisan publications, left and right, that are less opaque about their funding. But they too are a deviation from traditional local news, and not all readers will be aware of small print disclosing the partisan backing.[48] And this doesn't even take into account all the fake news and fake news outlets that foreign adversaries like Russia, China, and Iran have planted, but that's more in the sphere of political and international affairs—though health and vaccination news is not immune.⁴⁹

"Slime" sites tell readers that government is failing, incompetent, or corrupt, and the conservative ideology creeps into health coverage. For instance, a purported news release from a local hospital on one Florida site appeared to be a fake—that release didn't appear anywhere in the hospital's own archive of press statements. The hospital "release," posted on the news site in the fall of 2022 as COVID-19 cases ticked up again, told readers how to tell whether they had a cold, the flu, or pneumonia. COVID-19 didn't make the list, creating the impression that it was no longer (or had never been) a problem. Exploring further on the web as we researched this book, we discovered that a hospital did in fact issue that release. But not the local hospital that the news site had attributed it to. And even more misleading, the release had been disseminated two and a half years earlier, in January 2020. Of course, it didn't mention the coronavirus or tell people what to watch for or how to protect themselves. It was written just as the first cases of what would become the pandemic were emerging in China, and the virus had not been identified in the United States. That particular pink slime site, the *Apopka Times*, vanished from the web at some point after our initial search, but plenty of others remained.⁵⁰

In at least a few documented cases, print versions of biased pseudo-sites appeared in people's mailboxes right before the 2022 elections. They were traced to the same interlocking conservative organizations behind the digital sites.⁵¹

In other communities, local corporations and business interests are taking advantage of the decline in local news. For instance, Florida Power and Light, a utility that was under scathing criticism at the time, secretly took over a news site called the Capitolist. The *Miami Herald*, in a series of articles published in the summer of 2022, revealed the transactions and shell companies that ran the "newspaper," and documented how private communications consultants working for Florida Power and Light screened the articles, attempting to create an environment where the utility could push back against regulators and critics and out-of-state government.[52] A subsequent award-winning investigation by National Public Radio and Floodlight, a nonprofit environmental news cooperative, found that both the Florida power company and Alabama Power were part of a much larger project that involved undisclosed payments to several local news outlets that were favorable to the utility companies—whose agendas did not include fighting climate change that threatens human health.[53]

Still other fake news sites are covers for criminal activity. In a practice known as typosquatting or brandjacking, these sites use URLs that are similar to those of legitimate media, exploiting the typos people make when they search for domains and then scooping up their data. It's fake news but with a monetary, not ideological, motive. For example, one fake news site, abcnews.com.co—created to fool people looking for abcnews.com—ran a story claiming that people were being paid to protest at Donald Trump's rallies. The author of the fiction told *The Washington Post* he earned $10,000 monthly from advertisements on his sites.[54]

And in at least one case, a politician, then–Arizona independent Senator Kyrsten Sinema, ran campaign ads on a Facebook page called "The Desert Recap" designed to look like local news. Though it did include a disclaimer (for a reader who looked closely enough), the ads were dressed up to look like news reports on her achievements, *The Daily Beast* reported in August 2022.[55]

Consequences for Health

In this environment, health reporting is uneven at best, as papers struggle to survive with fewer staff and tighter budgets. The consequences for health are real and growing.

Less Awareness

Where there are fewer local journalists, there is less understanding of key health issues facing communities. There is less attention to increases in rabies, sexually transmitted diseases, or contaminated water. There are fewer opportunities to draw attention to low rates of immunization, smoking cessation, or hypertension control. Reporting on gun policy—emphasizing the horrific mass shootings and not adequately or accurately reporting on the daily violence in many communities—creates an inaccurate public perception of risks and harms, as organizations like the Philadelphia Center for Gun Violence Reporting have shown.[56] Despite the heightened awareness of the mental health and suicide crisis in the country, there's still a lot of misunderstanding about mental illness itself, perpetuating stigma and creating barriers to care.

As one California mental health activist pointed out, coverage of that state's Care Act—a contested new program that can in some cases mandate care for seriously mentally ill people without their consent—tended to focus on the political debate over coercion and civil rights, sometimes without even quoting a single psychiatrist in the story.[57] They tended to lump all mental illnesses together, not explaining what is different about serious brain diseases like schizophrenia or noting that those who do not voluntarily get treatment—because the nature of the disease often means they don't recognize that they need treatment—risk ending up incarcerated or homeless. "I don't want to diss the reporters because I know how complex the issues are in this particular topic with mental illness, serious brain diseases," the California mental health activist said. But she added, "Our politics and policies have not kept up with the science of the illness and we're not treating them like an illness."[58] Her critique doesn't mean California's approach is necessarily a step forward. It just means that the coverage, in this advocate's eyes at least, is too incomplete to allow for truly informed public debate.

More Errors

The challenges facing local news are not just challenges of omission or lack of coverage. They're also problems of poor journalism—journalism pursued on the cheap, with less training, fewer experienced editors, and less developed judgment. That leads to problems like a small Colorado paper referring to a controversial "experimental" medication abortion reversal treatment—the phrase "experimental" implies it's being studied and might work—without explaining until deep down into a fairly long story that it's not so much "experimental" as discredited.[59] The constant search for "eyeballs" and "clicks"—that is, readers or viewers or listeners—can also encourage splashy or sensational headlines that aren't 100 percent accurate.

Reporters at local papers, who tend to be starting out in their careers, just can't develop expertise if they are covering half a dozen or more beats—and a thinning of the editing ranks means they don't have guides and mentors. So they get things wrong—outright wrong, or wrong in terms of weight and emphasis. Even small mistakes, of fact or emphasis, can confuse the public, and even small errors about health can cause outright harm. A small-town paper covering a fight over a proposal to tax e-cigarettes probably shouldn't rely on the owner of a local vaping shop as the principal voice in a story, with a pro forma local smoking cessation expert given a few perfunctory lines toward the bottom.[60]

Beyond content errors, inexperienced and overburdened reporters can also make mistakes of emphasis. If they don't know whether something is new and significant, and if they don't have a more seasoned editor or colleague to weigh in, they may end up giving weight to something that's not really important. On the flip side, they miss things that their readers really should know to protect themselves and their loved ones, or to support healthy public policies. Frustrated public officials may attribute these errors to laziness or stupidity, when the actual culprit a tendency in newsrooms to ask reporters to do too much too quickly, without good sources to rely on for quick checks. (Savvy public health officials reach out to these reporters to become sources—and resources.)

Gaps in reporting matter, and they became famous, or infamous, during the debate over the Affordable Care Act (ACA), otherwise known as Obamacare. The term "misinformation" wasn't used as much back then, but the lack of expertise was evidence. The Republicans wanted to kill the health legislation, so they and allies in the media distorted it and amplified its flaws. The demonization didn't require a lot of technical precision. It fell on the Democrats to explain and defend a law that was big and complicated with a lot of moving parts—and they didn't do a very good job. Reporters without deep understanding often oversimplified it, either boiling it down to an easier-to-understand political battle or describing its complicated provisions in ways that highlighted the flaws and buried—or outright omitted—the benefits.

From the passage of the law in 2010 through the early years of enrollment and on through the fight over "repeal and replace," there were countless negative stories about Obamacare. Many focused on the unpopular individual mandate, without mentioning how many people were exempt from it, or how broad the exemptions were. Ditto for the avalanche of stories about how unaffordable ACA health insurance premiums were, without mentioning the subsidies millions of Americans could get.[61] In fact, one study found that even in a subset of local television stories in 2013–2014 that did focus at least somewhat on the coverage provisions, only a measly 7 percent even mentioned the existence of subsidies to make care affordable.[62] That doesn't mean reporters should have ignored the controversy; Obamacare was an animating force in American politics and the controversy affected elections for the better part of a decade. It does mean reporters should have covered it more fully and accurately—and not, as one paper in Idaho did, write stories about how expensive and terrible the law was, because local insurance brokers said so.[63]

Even three or four years into the ACA, as the Republicans pumped up their repeal campaign after Trump's 2016 election, coverage around the open enrollment season remained flawed. "Newspapers passed along GOP talking points about 'death spirals' and an Obamacare collapse, or failed to explain the often incorrect recommendations from state insurance department officials," a critique in the *Columbia*

Journalism Review found. "And too many newsrooms passed along that classic and trite consumer line—'shop around'—without saying how people should do that."[64]

This coverage not only fueled the decade-long political warfare, it didn't give people what they needed to know about their own insurance options, their own financial protection, or their own ability to take care of themselves and their loved ones if someone got sick. Even several years into the ACA, millions of eligible people didn't even bother "window-shopping" on the health exchange portals for insurance, convinced that it was unaffordable. A Commonwealth Fund survey in 2018 found that, with an estimated 30.4 million people still uninsured, two-thirds had not even gone to the online marketplaces to look at their coverage choices. One-third of them said they didn't think insurance would be affordable. Yet almost half of the uninsured adult population may have been eligible for subsidies or expanded Medicaid.[65]

With the rise of social media, errors in local journalism do not just blow down the street with yesterday's news. Harmful myths, or outright lies, jump from the "respectable" and "objective" local TV or radio station onto social media—where some reporter from another overworked and underresourced TV station will see them, believe they are reliable, and put them on the air. It is a dangerous cycle that can be repeated again and again. This is particularly worrisome as people often have more trust in local television for health news than in national outlets; a Knight Foundation survey confirmed this was true during the pandemic.[66] And the increasing use of artificial intelligence can add to the error recycling. Once erroneous information is ingested by AI, it pops up again and again.

More False Equivalence

Presenting both sides, or multiple sides, of a story is generally a good thing; fairness, balance, and completion are the essence of what reporters are supposed to do. At the same time, when evidence, facts, and science clearly support one side of a debate, journalists should make that clear too. For instance, a tiny paper in Brigham City, Utah, called the *Box Elder News Journal* published several stories in which local dentists and dental organizations explained the benefits of fluoride. "Orthodontist Calls on Voters to Keep Fluoride," was one headline.[67] The paper appropriately put the debate on its opinion pages to present "both sides" of a 2023 ballot initiative to stop fluoridating the town's water. The effort to remove fluoride failed.

False equivalence, also known as "both sidesism" or "whataboutism," is the act of putting on equal footing perspectives with vastly different factual bases. In the worst-case scenario, such journalism inadvertently legitimizes falsehood in the name of "balance." Coverage of climate change and its threats to human health is a good example. Coverage has been infused with the voices of science skeptics, some funded by the fossil fuel industry, determined to cast doubt over the deepening scientific consensus that the planet is warming.[68] Abortion is another example. As a small study, based on interviews with self-identified feminist or progressive journalists, in the journal *Contraception* found, reporters are often pressed to present "both sides" on abortion—not about the political, moral, and religious arguments, which can be hard to bridge, but about the scientific and medical facts. The scientific facts about the physical safety of terminating a pregnancy are well established, but stories often overstate risks or contain inaccurate information about things like mental illness or infertility after an abortion. Some of the journalists who wrote these stories have described how their editors didn't really understand the facts about abortion; one recounted that her editor seemed to think it was akin to a C-section.[69]

With the proper context, it may be fine for an article or report to note that there is dissent. After all, the dissenters and deniers can shape—or block—climate policy. Or water fluoridation. Or vaccine mandates. Or access to legal abortion. But an article noting the opinions of climate change skeptics should also make crystal clear the breadth and depth of the scientific consensus on climate. (Or fluoridation. Or vaccines. Or abortion.) Fact and denial of fact are not on equal footing. In our polarized society, this balance is harder to strike than it should be. At least one local TV meteorologist, Chris Gloninger, received death threats in response to his factual reporting linking extreme weather and climate change. The station, a CBS affiliate in Des Moines, Iowa, wanted him to dial his coverage down, according to an Associated Press report. Gloninger ended up quitting his job and leaving town. He left journalism too, taking a job with an environmental consulting organization.[70]

False equivalence may be more likely when a brand-new threat emerges—HIV back in the 1980s, and more recently Zika, Ebola, or SARS and later its pandemic-causing cousin SARS-CoV-2. When something scary and new bursts onto the scene, there may be limited expertise and clarity, particularly in the local news universe. When the right answers are not immediately clear and available, bad reporting can make things worse for the public. The cautious scientific, medical, or public health voices may be saying, "We don't know for sure." The unreliable science-denying voices may come across as more certain and definitive. As a new crisis unfolds, reporters are at risk for elevating the wrong voices and depicting science as unreliable or mercurial, rather than as a step-by-step process. This is an area where all the misinformation and disinformation on social media, which we saw in the case of Keith Smith (the patient who died while taking ivermectin), and discuss in chapter 3, can seep into bad local reporting.

Vaccination, of course, has been a fertile field of false equivalence for years, particularly after the incorrect, ultimately retracted, but stubbornly persistent study in the medical journal *Lancet* linking vaccination and autism. Years before COVID-19 emerged, a local Philadelphia TV station segment on a new meningitis B vaccine included both Paul Offit, the internationally renowned director of the Vaccine Education Center at Children's Hospital of Philadelphia and a world-renowned expert in virology and immunology, and Sherri Tenpenny, a vaccine critic who, during the pandemic, would achieve a kind of notoriety for her claim that the COVID-19 shots make people magnetic.

"What bothers us as scientists," Offit told a health journalism conference in 2014, "is that you told 'two sides' of this story when, frankly, only one side is supported by the science." He characterized this habit of journalists as "false balance."[71]

"I don't see that as informing the public. I see it as misinforming the public," Offit added. And misinformation means people can make bad decisions, decisions that can harm their health or the health of their family.[72]

False equivalence ran rampant during the pandemic. From red Florida to blue California, many local TV stations gave local physicians free airtime—even if they were evangelizing conspiracy theories about vaccines and unfounded promises of "cures" like ivermectin—without reporting their ties to discredited groups like America's Frontline Doctors or the Children's Health Defense organization, the nonprofit that Robert F. Kennedy Jr. chaired before being tapped as Trump's HHS secretary in 2025.[73]

More Distrust

Public officials who are doing their best to communicate well can be undermined by poor journalism. It is an axiom of good public health communication to, in the words of former Surgeon General Jerome Adams, "tell them what you know, tell them what you don't know and tell them how you [are going] to find out." He added, "It sounds simple but it's hard to do, and it's really hard to do in a world of communication by tweets and then headlines."[74] Instead of helping readers and viewers understand that knowledge will evolve and change, underresourced local journalists may puff up initial announcements in ways that raise hopes and then create bitter disappointments when circumstances change. It's easy to rely on lightly rewritten press releases, produced by PR companies that get paid to earn news coverage. Reputable research institutions too have incentives to try to get attention for their work, including by hailing preliminary lab findings as "breakthroughs." Research done on cells or even in mice is one step on a long path toward developing drugs and treatment—and most of these "breakthroughs" that make headlines never actually come to fruition.

But when such breakthroughs don't pan out, the result can be disillusionment and distrust. Sometimes journalists—feeling betrayed—can exacerbate this problem by portraying health officials who are reporting changes in science as "flip-floppers" or even liars.

Less Accountability

The decline of local news also means scantier coverage of what public officials are doing to address major health challenges. A recent example is the sporadic coverage of how states and localities are spending proceeds from opioid litigation. An investigation found major gaps in transparency in the groups set up to spend these funds; without enterprising local reporters, it may be difficult to assess whether the money is supporting promising work or discredited programs that might actually make things worse.[75]

Local news outlets undertake fewer investigations into health care and public health trends and challenges, into the response to those challenges, and into interference with that response. Maybe a paper will run a wire story about a national trend, but local outlets don't necessarily dive in, beyond rewriting press releases, or ask the key questions about overdose deaths, homicides, chronic disease, gun violence, access to food, the link between health and lack of housing, or access to care. Attention to these problems can lead to change; ignoring them makes them worse.

Even when reporters do turn to a health problem, they do not necessarily scrutinize the nature of the response. Are health officials on top of key data, directing resources to urgent issues? Or are they largely unaware, unable to muster a response to help communities in need? Are they communicating in ways that the public can understand—and in ways that engender trust? Without good local reporting, it is difficult for the public to hold officials accountable for their actions and inactions, whether it's a response to a pandemic or oversight of a government health program.

In 2018, *The Dallas Morning News* investigated for-profit Medicaid plans in an example of accountability in action. The reporting prompted state legislators to hold hearings into the harm done to very sick and fragile children and disabled adults. Both Democratic and Republican lawmakers introduced bills to address the problem, and a bipartisan package was enacted.[76] And the Texas agency with oversight of Medicaid announced it would hire about 100 new regulators—including nurses to pay home visits to vulnerable patients.[77] But—and this often happens as good reporters seek larger platforms—both the reporters who led the investigation moved on to major national outlets, ProPublica and *The New York Times*. Neither is still engaged primarily in local news.

Accountability isn't just important for health officials; it's important for the elected leaders who appoint and oversee health officials. During the pandemic, many turned against public health—firing public health officers or forcing them to quit or retire. Many stood silent while health officials endured severe harassment and death threats against them and their families. Online or in public meetings, people advocated hangings, shootings, and even the gas chamber for public health officials who backed mask or vaccine mandates and other pandemic mitigation steps.[78]

In Michigan—where Governor Gretchen Whitmer was the intended victim of a kidnapping and murder plot because of her pandemic public health policies—at least eight local health officers and nine medical directors had quit or taken retirement about a year and a half after the pandemic started.[79] In Riverside County, California, health officer Cameron Kaiser was subject to an intense backlash and ugly threats after he put in strict restrictions on social gatherings early in the pandemic. A fake Twitter account depicted him with a Hitler mustache. Rather than support him, county officials fired him.[80] Conversely, in Idaho a pathologist who prescribed ivermectin and who called vaccination "needle rape" was named to the sole physician seat on the state's largest regional public health agency.[81] State legislatures also enacted numerous restrictions on public health officials' ability to do their jobs, leaving the country more vulnerable in the next public health emergency.[82]

Inadequate local news coverage left many citizens unaware of these events. The failure to report fully on what happened will make it harder to hire good people and raises the risk that elected officials will undermine the essential work of public health officials when the inevitable next crisis lands on our doors.

Fighting to Save Local News

Not every small-town paper is headed for extinction. Traditional advertising and revenue sources may have failed, but readers, viewers, and listeners still want news. A number of nonprofit initiatives have been investing in efforts to fortify and sustain local news outlets; others are backing the new start-ups we'll explore in chapters 4 and 5. The National Trust for Local News, for instance, has acquired economically struggling small community papers in several states and is helping them survive and thrive on a new nonprofit business basis.[83] With help from the MacArthur Foundation (best known for its "genius grants"), another new organization called Press Forward brought together a score of charitable organizations, many with local roots, to put more than $500 million in local news in 2023.[84] Organizations like Report for America (an offshoot of the Ground Truth Project, which helps emerging journalists globally) find talented young journalists and match them up with local newsrooms for two- to three-year stints, with Report for America paying half their salaries and helping the host paper raise a portion of the other half. (The host paper also contributes.)[85] Other foundations are enabling the emerging nonprofit sector discussed in chapter 4.

Some outlets come up with their own solutions. And what they accomplish is a reminder of what the news deserts have lost.

The Seattle Times, which has the advantage of being the hometown paper for a number of very wealthy tech entrepreneurs engaged in philanthropy, created an investigative journalism fund for a large reporting team. It also raised money for several smaller policy reporting initiatives, including a four-person mental health unit supported by philanthropies such as the Ballmer Group. The Seattle paper, like others relying on outside donations, maintains full editorial control. The mental health team is bigger than the entire health reporting units at comparably sized newspapers. And the funding means it can dig deep and take time on stories. Free from the clickbait pressures and able to stop, think, and explore, they can approach the topic in a way that reporters elsewhere cannot.[86]

Hannah Furfaro is one of the two full-time reporters on the *Seattle Times* mental health unit. She started out in journalism about 15 years ago at a small paper in Iowa and experienced a lot of the same frustrations as other reporters with big ideas in a shrinking media world. She moved on, doing more science writing along the way. By 2017, she was on staff at *Spectrum*, a publication that covers autism and related disorders. In 2019, she went to the Seattle paper.

"I'm very fortunate being on this team. In some ways we're freed from this drumbeat of the news cycle. I get to do a lot of enterprise and investigative reporting," she said. With her background in science and health, she can do stories about innovation and treatment, including some "local angle" coverage of the work coming out of the Seattle-based University of Washington. But she's also done powerful stories about people experiencing mental illness, and the system that fails them.[87]

One multipart series that meant a great deal to her focused on young people with psychiatric conditions. "There are few inpatient psychiatric beds for kids in Washington, and there's also really poor access to outpatient care," she said. "Oftentimes it [the care] is actually good but the wait lists are long. So what happens is kids just don't get care, and they wind up in crisis."[88]

She told the stories of "youths who end up actually living in emergency departments or on medical floors [of hospitals] waiting for appropriate psychiatric care. These are kids, you know, who might be experiencing suicidal thoughts or self harming, or in a state of psychosis or catatonia. The E.R., as you might imagine, is basically the absolute worst place you could be if you're in that state of mind." She also did a story on how more and more kids are placed in restraints, which is disturbing not just for the young patients and their families but for the health workers caring for them."[89] In a more typical newsroom, without the additional philanthropic supports *The Seattle Times* receives, Furfaro "definitely would not have been able, been afforded the time or resources to do a series like this."[90]

Her work did more than draw attention to kids in crisis. It prompted Washington State to change its laws, providing better and more appropriate care to these children and adolescents stuck in hospitals.[91]

In Charleston, South Carolina—a community that doesn't have a lot in common with Seattle, economically, politically, or culturally—another local newspaper with a proud tradition of accountability reporting decided it needed to do something different. Once known for its fierce segregationist stance, *The Post and Courier* had over the decades evolved into a publication known for its investigative work and enterprise reporting. But like many of its peers, the newspaper found that its financial model for sustaining its journalism was increasingly vulnerable. Print subscribers migrated to digital platforms, advertisers migrated to Google and Facebook, and internet sources killed once lucrative classified advertising. About 80 cents of every dollar of advertising revenue was being lost to ads on Facebook, Google, and other internet sites. Subscriptions didn't fill the gap.

Rather than give up the kind of reporting that made them want to come to work every day, editors began a fundraising campaign, creating a philanthropic-backed arm to support investigative work. The paper quickly surpassed its own expectations, raising more than $1 million.[92] "Our goal was to raise $100,000 in 100 days, and we raised half a million in a couple of months," said *Post and Courier* senior projects reporter Tony Bartelme, who has been involved with the endeavor from the start.[93]

And what's more, *The Post and Courier* spread a protective umbrella over other local news outlets as well. In a project called "Uncovered"—the name refers to both stories that hadn't been told and the wrongdoing that hadn't been exposed—the paper invited local journalists in more than 17 communities to team up with six *Post and Courier* reporters to "shine the brightest light possible on conduct that is holding our state back, benefitting the few at the expense of the many."[94]

"Corruption has flourished in South Carolina as newspapers close and shrink, creating news deserts and ghost papers across the Palmetto State," *The Post and Courier* said in its call for partners. "It's part of a national trend that has deprived hundreds of communities of a vital watchdog of taxpayer dollars and democracy."[95] All the stories were published in both *The Post and Courier* and the community outlets, available without a subscription. The result was a stream of revelations, some about corruption, some about health and safety (and some about both).[96] "Uncovered" revealed utility commissioners enjoying wine tastings, zip lines, and four-star retreats at ratepayers' expense.[97] It found a superintendent who lived in housing for teachers, as well as "scores" of public officials who had failed to pay fines for violating the state's ethic laws.[98] The reporters also discovered a failure to investigate a rape allegation against a sheriff, toxic mold spreading in college dorms, and corruption in a local coroner's office.[99] In one of the worst examples, the reporters found nasty drinking water that resulted from broken pumps, weed killer and ant poison near wells, and sludge coating water tanks.[100]

If anyone wanted proof that local journalism matters, that its disappearance harms, "Uncovered" fills the bill.

"We leverage our investigative resources with their on-the-ground knowledge, and then work together in whatever way works for everybody," said Bartelme, describing the partnerships with reporters in smaller towns, including some who focus on Black and Latino communities. "And that's sort of the key to success. Some of these local journalists just don't have time or the experience to do—or money to do—deep dives. And if they don't have the time, then we sort of just take the lead, but it's a very collaborative experience. And the collaboration has worked because it's loose and respects the independence and differing needs of our partners."[101]

Bartelme said the paper has gotten queries about "Uncovered" from a lot of other small newspapers—as far away as Pakistan—although no one had yet quite replicated it. Meanwhile, building on "Uncovered," which is ongoing, *The Post and Courier* created another community-funded initiative called "Rising Waters" to document the local impact of climate change.[102] The paper built new databases to identify vulnerable areas and homes, and had floodwaters analyzed for fecal contamination, an underappreciated threat to public health. "We waited for one of those increasingly common downpours and tidal floods to make a mess of things. When they did, we embedded our deeply reported climate science pieces into breaking stories," he wrote in an essay for the American Association for the Advancement of Science.[103]

The aim was to "cover climate change as the breaking story that it truly is—but with more depth and when the effects were as visceral as the chaos swirling through readers' yards."[104] It's had an impact; new policies have been put into effect, including a $10 million plan to protect the medical district in Charleston.

"Will the model we used for 'Uncovered' work for other topics, such as climate change and other complex science-based topics?" he wrote. "We think so. When a hurricane hits, why not tap the Uncovered network to create a much more robust region-wide story? Why not share the contextual pieces about climate change? A 'Rising Waters 2.0.'"[105]

In some ways, Bartelme's career path recalls that of Eric Eyre—and not just because they both fell in love with newspapers in towns named Charleston. Both love being close to their community, even as their reporting accolades have opened other career possibilities. (Eyre won the Pulitzer; Bartelme is a rare four-time finalist.) But Bartelme stayed in his Charleston for some 30 years. Eyre also stayed in his Charleston, for nearly 25 years, finding other reporting and writing outlets after leaving the *Gazette-Mail*. Both are committed to local news, to public health, to ambitious reporting, to holding those in power accountable to the people who gave them that power.

That longevity is "unusual," said Bartelme. "But that's sort of part of our successes, that we've been here for a long time. We've had opportunities to go elsewhere, but we just kind of like it here."[106]

"Uncovered" provides reassurance that the promise of local journalism remains strong, even as its very existence is at stake in so much of the country. But among the headwinds complicating its resurgence is the loss of support from the national level. As the next chapter shows, the media crisis—and the crisis in coverage essential to Americans' good health—extends to the national news sources that used to highlight and supplement local coverage. The polarization, conflict, and outrage now so dominant in society at large are mirrored in the national media—and that's not good for our information environment, or for our health.

• CHAPTER 2

The Fracturing of National News

The coronavirus pandemic was Ricardo Alonso-Zaldivar's last big story.

Over a career that spanned decades, Alonso-Zaldivar had worked for, among other places, the now-defunct Knight Ridder chain of midsize city papers gobbled up in corporate mergers, and for the *Los Angeles Times*, before its purchase by controversial biotech billionaire Patrick Soon-Shiong. In 43 years in the news business, until his retirement in May 2022, he covered a variety of political and policy stories, including a lot of health, on and off Capitol Hill. Starting in 2008, he covered health for the Associated Press, first focusing on the US Food and Drug Administration and then shifting more to health policy as the debate over the Affordable Care Act (ACA) intensified after Barack Obama took office in 2009.

The wire services are a backbone of national news coverage. Small local papers like those featured in chapter 1 regularly use the wires, which reach all 50 states and most of the globe, to give their readers some national news. Large papers use it to fill gaps in their own coverage, particularly where budget woes similar to those constraining local news have shuttered bureaus and cut staff. Editors use the wires to get a sense of what's going on in the world on any given day and how they may want to deploy their own reporters. In this way, wire service dispatches and daily news advisories have helped set the agenda and tone for newsrooms nationwide.

During the busy last 15 years of his career, Alonso-Zaldivar's Associated Press stories helped guide the health beat, particularly his reports on the passage of the ACA, its clumsy implementation, and the failed Republican crusade to repeal it. When a mysterious virus broke out in China, it was, as he recalled, "all hands on deck."[1] Like many other policy reporters well versed in Medicare policy or fights over regulation or the workings of the Food and Drug Administration, Alonso-Zaldivar suddenly had to learn to cover a pandemic.

He understood the political games of Washington, the ways that health care affected voters and politics. He was also a meticulous reporter who paid attention to the small print, to the details of legislative proposals and budgets and laws. He understood that there are legitimate, and important, debates about the role of government in health care, about how much public money should be spent and how and on whom. "It has become very, very, very politicized," he said.

> But it was always going to be political for two reasons. One reason, which has kind of faded [from news coverage], is the enormous cost. Long-term cost-wise, it's the biggest challenge for the federal government. The other reason, which is closer to the flashpoint of politics, is because it has to do with the role of government in people's private lives. So for those two reasons, health care's always going to be political. And sure you have to appreciate that and cover it with gusto.[2]

But he also understood that on the health care beat, politics wasn't the only story.

"You've got to cover the daily story, whatever that is," he recalled. "But beyond that . . . your focus should be on how health care affects people. How health care decisions in Washington affect people." A debate over single-payer care may dominate a Democratic primary for a season, but it's important to explain what it would mean for people, not just candidates. "I liked doing stories that try to explain how decisions made on behalf of the American people affect us."[3]

Now retired, and with the benefit of hindsight, Alonso-Zaldivar looks back at all the hoopla and fighting about things like the Obamacare individual mandate, and wonders whether the public would have been better served by more reporting on Medicare, which covers all Americans starting at age 65, and Medicaid, a safety net for tens of millions of low-income Americans, including children.

> All Americans are affected by Medicare—as taxpayers, as future beneficiaries, as family members of beneficiaries. And Medicaid is for the most vulnerable—it's becoming the "National Health Program" for children, for low-income people. And a lot of those things cut across all the states. . . . If I had my druthers, we'd spend more time covering those things. We do a pretty good job of covering the buzz in the health care policy debates, but we neglect the old dictum that journalists are taught to follow the money, and the money is in those two entitlement programs, Medicare and Medicaid.[4]

Health care isn't always the hottest story in DC, but Alonso-Zaldivar consistently had editors, at all his jobs, who recognized that it always mattered. "I was lucky, year in and year out and in different organizations, to work for editors who were interested."[5] He had their support to chase the stories he thought were important.

But while he was able to do substantive work on so many aspects of health and public health, he recognized that the national media was changing. His Associated Press editors might have given him the time and space to work on health stories he thought were worthwhile, but that didn't mean his stories, no matter how deeply reported and well crafted, always got a lot of play in papers across the country when health care wasn't "hot" politically. Some outlets would prioritize it and then drop it until it heated up again; others would emphasize the politics over the policy. He didn't leave reporting because of those national trends; he left because it was the right moment, for him and his family, to retire after a distinguished 43-year run. But the health reporters still on the beat are operating in a world that makes the possibility of a career like his increasingly unlikely.[6]

The Battlefield

Many of us share a mental image of the United States during the Depression and the Second World War: families huddled closely around their radios, escaping into comedies or dramas, or leaning into the reassuring voice of Franklin Roosevelt. A generation later, it was television. With three commercial networks, and later PBS, the viewing audience of that era similarly shared a common national narrative—albeit one that was shaped by a small number of largely white and male reporters and network executives. While local papers fostered closeness to our communities, radio and TV allowed us to share common experiences with our country and the broader world.

Now, they divide us.

Talking heads. Strategists. Commentators. Horse races. Inside baseball. Polls, polls, and more polls.

That's become the bulk of national news coverage, with stories like those that Alonso-Zaldivar used to write becoming vanishingly rare. Even the top three or four daily newspapers—which still do employ health reporters—have more than their share of horse-race reporting, a hyperfocus on who is up and who is down, strategy over substance. Policy gets short shrift, or is just not done very well. Often, policy reporting has begun to mirror the horse-race style of reporting, where the focus, as media critic Jay Rosen has pointed out, is too often on the odds, not the stakes.[7]

While the big national news outlets aren't as endangered as the small local newspapers described in the previous chapter, they too have gone through waves of layoffs and buyouts and shrinkage as they seek to adapt to the new digital landscape that has siphoned off subscribers and squeezed traditional sources of revenue. A handful have been purchased by billionaires, notably the *Los Angeles Times*, as noted earlier, and *The Washington Post*, owned by Amazon founder Jeff Bezos. Their involvement has not guaranteed strong economic returns, but it has raised concerns about whether the commingling of media and wealth best serves democracy.[8]

The contribution of the national media to political conflict has heightened in recent decades. The introduction of broadcast media—radio in the 1920s and 1930s and television in the 1940s and 1950s, both of which qualify as what we'd now call "disruptive" technology—actually corresponded with decreased partisanship, according to research from Harvard Kennedy School scholars Filipe Campante and Daniel Hojman.[9]

"There is 'robust evidence' that the introduction of broadcast TV decreased the polarization in Congress," Campante and Hojman wrote. "More precisely, places where TV was introduced earlier displayed a decrease in different measures of the extremism of their representatives, relative to late coming places."[10] Not only were there only three networks in those days—and local radio consolidated quickly into ownership by four big networks—but what each network reported didn't differ all that much (and the faces on camera, and most of the decision makers behind them, were white and male). They were the mainstream media, and in their wake was mainstream thinking. The data on early radio are less abundant than TV, but they point to a similar homogenizing influence.

That is no longer the case. During the Reagan administration, the Federal Communications Commission repealed what was called the Fairness Doctrine. This policy had required TV stations to provide equivalent coverage to different sides, to make sure a variety of viewpoints on an issue were aired. After its repeal, news outlets may still have had the moral obligation to delve into multiple facets of a complex policy debate, but they no longer had the legal requirement.

The repeal enabled talk radio to flourish, and conservative voices found a footing and echo chamber there while the more liberal voices who tried to establish a presence on talk radio foundered or remained relatively small. Talk radio helped pave the way for polarized cable television news with the politically conservative Fox News and later for left-leaning coverage at stations like MSNBC. They now had "the freedom to express strong opinions and views without fear of regulatory reprisal," according to an approving Heritage Foundation assessment of the post–Fairness Doctrine world.[11] Fox tapped into long-simmering conservative beliefs that the mainstream media had a liberal bias and did not serve those on the right. The polarization, on left and right, was also part of the emerging business model. In an era of proliferating TV choices, available on cable 24/7, outlets needed to appeal to, attract, and maintain viewers who were no longer restricted to a half hour of broadcast news at the dinner hour. The partisanship, the tribalism, became the brand.

In 2016, the election year that saw Donald Trump ascend, these forces coalesced. Back in 2007 and 2008, when health policy was a major thread in both the Democratic presidential primary race and the general election, it didn't dominate coverage, according to a Pew Research Center analysis. It represented less than 1 percent of campaign-related news.[12] There was a whole lot more coverage of diseases and illnesses, particularly cancer.

Fast-forward to 2016. Pew didn't conduct a similar health coverage survey during that presidential election cycle, but the media-monitoring *Tyndall Report* did track overall policy coverage until the final few weeks of the campaign. It found that the three major broadcast nightly news programs during that campaign season spent a total of just 32 minutes covering *all* policy issues—not just health. And that was mostly foreign policy and security. This was amid hours and hours of coverage of which candidates were up or down, Andrew Tyndall found.[13] That was far less policy news than prior election seasons, although the downward slide had already begun by 2012. The 2016 campaign was admittedly not a policy-heavy season. Trump wasn't running as a man with a policy plan; he was starring in his one-man show of political theater.

It was his opponent, Hillary Clinton, who was known as the queen of policy, but her expertise became something to mock rather than analyze. She received less overall coverage than Trump—and, for long periods of time, more negative coverage than Trump.[14] "Both Hillary Clinton and Donald Trump received coverage that was overwhelmingly negative in tone and extremely light on policy"—and while neither got much policy coverage, she got less than he did, the Shorenstein Center on Media, Politics and Public Policy concluded in a series of studies entitled "The Press Failed the Voters."[15]

With a pandemic raging, and the economy in disarray, 2020 coverage was only a smidgen better from a policy perspective. A Shorenstein Center follow-up study of the 2020 campaign, using CBS weekday evening news as a stand-in for all mainstream TV versus Fox News' evening newscast, found 10 percent of the time the *CBS Evening News* spent on Joe Biden was devoted to policy issues (other than COVID-19) versus 12 percent on the Fox program.[16]

Many factors contributed to Trump's rise, but the news media, particularly cable and network television that got a ratings (and therefore revenue) boost from wall-to-wall Trump coverage, played a role. Trump's candidacy, CBS CEO Leslie Moonves told a Morgan Stanley tech investment conference in 2016, "may not be good for America, but it's damn good for CBS." Moonves went on to say, "The money's rolling in and this is fun. This is going to be a very good year for us. . . . Bring it on, Donald. Keep going."[17] (Moonves later claimed he had been joking.)[18]

Tracking firm mediaQuant estimated that Trump got more than $5 billion in free mentions in media during the course of his campaign, more than Hillary Clinton, Bernie Sanders, and several of his Republican primary rivals combined. Indeed, he got so much free media—and had so much free time on cable TV to talk and talk unchecked—that the business publication *The Street* reported he spent far less than a typical candidate on advertising and the organizational campaign activities known as the "ground game."[19]

The fact that we live in an era of perpetual campaigning—positioning, polling, and fundraising for the next campaign starts the moment the votes are counted in the last one, if not before—means the political horse-race coverage isn't restricted to a season. It's incessant. And it can squeeze out substantive and sustained coverage of other public concerns.

That includes public health preparedness. Health care costs. Homelessness. Gun violence. Mental health. The heating and degradation of the planet. As the late *Washington Post* columnist David Broder said, what the country really needs from political and campaign coverage is a lot less horse race, and a lot more of a job application for governing.[20] But in the years after he made that observation, national news coverage would become even more unbalanced.

Polarized Networks

The explosion of cable news created a cornucopia of options. That made for a lot of airtime hours to fill. And increasingly the 24/7 news hole has been filled with opinion, punditry, and commentary—which is cheaper to produce than in-depth news reports.[21] That very bounty of choices created pressure on the media outlets. They had to compete to attract, and retain, a share of the audience; their financial viability depended on it. And since the market is more fragmented, they need to cultivate loyal and frequent viewers—"highly habituated users," as former Fox political editor Chris Stirewalt called them. Stirewalt bemoaned the consequences of this tilt in *Broken News: Why the Media Rage Machine Divides America and How to Fight Back*, the book he wrote after being fired by Fox for making election-night calls in 2020 that were accurate but not favorable to Trump.[22] Conflict, controversy, and a general splashiness was the way to hook viewers and keep them on the line.

A sorting began. The objectivity that had characterized US news for most of the 20th century began to break down, particularly on TV. It became more political, and more divisive. Viewers and listeners tuned in to the voice, or echo chamber, of their own tribe. Over time, major national broadcast outlets began to disseminate misinformation and disinformation, including about life-threatening health crises like the pandemic or climate change. Or they told charged stories, for instance about transgender athletes, which stirred up hatred and fear.[23] And we were primed for those hatreds and divisions. As communications scholar Dannagal Goldthwaite Young wrote in *Wrong: How Media, Politics, and Identity Drive Our Appetite for Misinformation*, Americans are divided into tribes, or what Young calls teams.[24] The Fox viewing team doesn't see Fox as biased; they see bias happening over on MSNBC, the station of choice for the other, untrustworthy team. And the reverse is true—at least for those who are still watching news, who haven't just changed the channel (or their streaming service) to movies or sports.

In a time of crisis, political divides and public health divides become indistinguishable. An unfortunate legacy of the coronavirus pandemic is that public health—which had been largely nonpartisan even as the fights over health insurance intensified—was politicized too in both right-wing media and social media. Experts advocating measures that were meant to save people's lives—even if they made mistakes or did not always communicate uncertainty well enough—were demonized, hounded, and threatened. Suspicion and distrust exacerbated the already severe shortage in the public health workforce.

Among cable stations, Fox dominates.[25] Researchers, including a team at the National Bureau of Economic Research, have tied watching Fox News with both COVID-19 vaccination status and how well people followed other self-protective and community protective mitigation steps, like masking or social distancing. Using mobility data from cell phones, the research team found that Fox viewers were less likely to follow social distancing recommendations and stay home during the shutdown in March and April 2020. The study did note that there's a chicken-and-egg question here and in other analyses of this type: Were people more skeptical of public health measures, sometimes known as mitigation, because they watched Fox? Or did they watch Fox because it reinforced their skepticism of mitigation?[26]

Tucker Carlson, in his heyday on Fox, was a leading voice in turning a section of the country against public health officials and vaccination, elevating misunderstandings and misinformation even though Fox News itself had a vaccine mandate. People opposed to vaccination may have tuned in to hear the latest rant against the public health establishment, while those turning on Fox for other reasons could easily have gained skepticism as a result.

"Regardless of the mechanism," the National Bureau of Economic Research report said, "Fox News' coverage of COVID-19 has renewed concerns about potential risks from exposure (short or long-term) to misinformation."[27]

The polarization is only deepening.

Fox News and media outlets further to the right have altered the playbook for national news coverage, including by leading a rise in commentary that is often more prevalent on the air than actual news. Left-leaning news sources such as MSNBC also fuel what Stirewalt calls the "Outrage Machine"—and what scholars of communication have called the "economy of attention." "To cultivate the kind of intense readers, viewers or listeners necessary to make the addiction model profitable, media companies need consumers to have strong feelings," Stirewalt wrote. "Fear, resentment and anger work wonders. It helps news outlets create deep emotional connections to users not just as users of a product but as members of the same tribe."[28] And that dynamic spilled out from politics into health once the brief moment of national unity around the newly emergent coronavirus was replaced by blame and deep, bitter divisions.

The media, of course, does not bear sole responsibility for the polarization in American politics. Other factors include gerrymandering, which has left electoral races to be fought over ideological purity in a primary, rather than pitting one party's worldview against the other in November. That propels extreme candidates more than centrists or consensus builders—and these candidates are often more extreme than the public, who are much more centrist on hot-button issues like gun regulation or Medicaid expansion or tobacco taxes than politicians. Winner-take-all presidential primaries, which catapulted Trump to the front of the pack even though his 2016 opponents collectively had more support, further fuel polarization. Generally, party lines have hardened. There are fewer moderates, fewer crossover votes, more toeing the party line. It is quite simply less civil, less genial, than it has been in decades.

But the national media, particularly those with clear ideological tilts, have encouraged and profited from the ensuing conflict—and in doing so, have made it worse.

The Pull of Polls

News outlets like doing polls and reporting on polls. These surveys are seen as relatively objective and reasonably scientific, and they help justify newsroom decisions about which candidates to cover heavily and which to more or less sideline. Polls are easily accessible to reporters—and some carry their outlet's brand, such as "the NBC / Wall Street Journal poll." And since there's such a constant stream of new and updated polls during elections, the findings "help news media transform elections, relatively slow-moving phenomena, into daily news."[29] The continuous focus on who is up and who is down only deepens the "horse-race" nature of political coverage.

What's more, polls can be wrong. When horse-race polls err, some candidates can get an illegitimate boost, supporting their fundraising and voter turnout. When polls about policy are off, there can be misunderstandings about the true nature of support for key actions or positions.

Subtle changes in how questions are phrased or ordered can skew results, and the complexity of policy itself makes it harder to measure where Americans stand. Political scientists Adam Berinsky of MIT and Michele Margolis, then at MIT, later at the University of Pennsylvania, found that a lot of people—particularly those with less education—answered "I don't know" on polls about the ACA, a complex topic. Probing further, they found a lot of nonrespondents or people who answered "I don't know" actually supported the ACA even in its early, wobbly years, meaning it was more popular than the doomsayer headlines touted. "The result," Berinsky and Margolis wrote, was that polls presented "an incomplete portrait of public opinion on the issue of health care in the United States."[30]

It's impossible to know (though tantalizing to wonder) whether a more accurate assessment of Obamacare's public support might have short-circuited a full decade of negative and often ill-informed news coverage and fruitless fights over repeal, when that time and energy might have gone to something more constructive, like making US health care work better. Or preparing for a pandemic.

Gotcha!

One hallmark of superficial political reporting in national news is "gotcha" stories. When candidates or officials make serious misstatements, or worse, it's necessary for reporters to document it and call it out. The same is true when candidates "flip-flop" out of cowardice, ignorance, or expediency.

But that real reporting is different from disparaging as a flip-flop a change of policy that's based on new data or a reassessment of a changing environment. Or from sensationalizing or exaggerating the gaffe of the day. There's a difference between noting and reporting on minor flubs and inconsistencies—like the muddling of a line in a stump speech or the mispronunciation of the name of a foreign leader—and elevating them so that they dominate the news cycle for days and drown out coverage and debate of the underlying issues. The focus on the gaffe of the day—another lap in the horse race—substitutes for the harder work of reporting on what this politician or official or civic leader proposes to do as a senator or representative or governor or president and how it will affect the American public.

That gotcha style has spilled into health coverage. A political reporter might see a changing stance on a public health issue as flip-flopping or even prevaricating. A health beat reporter is more likely to understand that it's just how science works. Knowledge is incremental and it changes. That reality gets terribly lost when a gotcha headline emphasizes a momentary "wrongness" or inconsistency, rather than emphasizing, "Oh, the science changed. We now know more and have updated our thinking." The media's failure to understand "what science is, how science works, and what good science looks like" means that the media itself contributes to the politicization of science and the undermining of public trust, said Richard Besser, the president and CEO of the Robert Wood Johnson Foundation, a former acting director of the Centers for Disease Control (CDC), and the chief health and medical editor at ABC for seven years. It's also damaging to trust, he said, if scientists oversell what they know.[31]

"One of the things that struck me time and time again during the pandemic is how the media contributed to a narrative that whenever public health guidance changed, it meant that public health didn't know what it was doing—rather than the opposite, that this is good," said Besser. "This is what you want to see, that as you learn more, the guidance changes." Besser also pointed to a "lack of sophistication and the need within a lot of media outlets for creating this sense of conflict rather than this sense of explanation, of learning."[32]

"Every change," Besser said, "became a failure rather than, 'Wow, public health is on the ball.'"[33]

Former Surgeon General Jerome Adams has spoken in public about how he felt ill-treated by the gotcha and clickbait trends in journalism. In an hour-long appearance at a health journalism conference in March 2023, he described with discernible bitterness ways in which he felt misportrayed. Headlines persistently referred to him as "Trump's" surgeon general, which he attributed to the tendency of newsrooms to use words that would make their stories appear more prominently when someone does a web search on a given topic. The word "Trump" generates more clicks, more eyeballs, and in Adams's his view, it diminished him, reducing him from a public health official to a political hack. Surgeon General Vivek Murthy, who was both Adams's predecessor and his successor, wasn't as consistently called "Obama's surgeon general" or "Biden's surgeon general."[34]

Adams said that having everything he said flagged as from "a Trump official" made it hard for him to communicate in crucial stages of the pandemic, when liberals didn't trust anyone linked to Trump and conservatives didn't trust anyone linked to public health. "I was giving them [the public] accurate information at the time but people were calling it misinformation because it was from Donald Trump's Surgeon General," he recalled. "We need to understand the biases that we carry."[35]

Health reporters tended to get things right, he said, and even local reporters (in communities that still had local reporters) tended to listen to his public health message without looking for political conflict. But too often, it was national political reporters setting the tone—and not in a useful way.

It is possible to criticize gotcha journalism and still believe strongly in accountability reporting. Holding accountable the people in positions of power, or those seeking power, whether in the public or private sector, is a fundamental role of journalism. That applies to how transportation officials deal with a toxic spill, how the National Institutes of Health communicate science, how the CDC carries out testing, how the administration rolls out a website to buy insurance, when a mayor sells for her own personal benefit thousands of dollars of her self-published children's book to health systems in her city, and whether a Department of Health and Human Services secretary improperly spends tax dollars on charter jets.

But good journalism, whether local or national, is more than trumpeting a "scoop" into what's gone wrong. Reporters aren't supposed to be cheerleaders. But not all accountability reporting has to be negative. Reporters can and should also look into ways of fixing what's gone wrong, or what's working and could be made to work even better.

All these forces of negativity—the cynicism, the negativity, the gotcha—which are now baked into journalistic DNA, have become pernicious. From the reporters' side, a degree of skepticism, sometimes even hostility, is inevitable and appropriate—up to a point. But excessive, context-free negativity becomes harmful. Why debate solutions when all problems are intractable and all experts are untrustworthy? A 2016 study found the ratio of negative to positive stories on immigration was five to one, stories about Muslims were negative six to one, and stories about both the ACA and the economy were negative two to one both in major national print outlets and on TV.[36] This negativity, about politics, about the economy, about health, becomes damaging.

"A healthy dose of negativity is unquestionably a good thing," Harvard media scholar Thomas Patterson wrote. "An incessant stream of criticism has a corrosive effect. It needlessly erodes trust in political leaders and institutions and undermines confidence in government and policy." That in turn leads to even more cynicism and apathy among the public, which has come to believe there are no solutions, to health care or other challenges, that problems will just last forever and ever.[37]

The Diminishing Policy Beat

The pandemic gave a big boost to health coverage for obvious reasons; as Alonso-Zaldivar noted, it was all hands on deck in US newsrooms to cover the mysterious new virus dominating coverage around the world. But even with this boost, policy coverage was relatively modest and quickly gave way to the political dimensions of the pandemic response. "The media coverage tends to entertain and outrage more than inform," according to Nicole Hemmer, a Vanderbilt historian who has written in particular about conservative media. "It amplifies our partisan instincts instead of our civic ones. None of this is good for American democracy."[38] But it can be good for the media. Controversy sells.

These imperatives have challenged the few national health reporters who remain. The handful of top national papers like *The New York Times*, *The Washington Post*, and *The Wall Street Journal* have multiple reporters covering health, as does National Public Radio (which also has a nonprofit partnership to cover local health news, described in chapter 4). And these top-tier health journalists have the capability of breaking critical stories and providing important explanatory reporting. *The Washington Post*, for instance, investigated what happens when doctors give bad advice (like "Don't wear a mask" and "Stock up on ivermectin") and how little state medical boards do to discipline them.[39] *The New York Times* explored why the United States was—and remains—so slow to improve indoor air and ventilation, despite everything we have learned about how it can slow the spread of respiratory infections.[40] *Politico* revealed how Trump administration political appointees engaged in unprecedented meddling with the CDC journal

Morbidity and Mortality Weekly Report to make it align with Trump's own upbeat but inaccurate messaging about COVID-19.[41] Earlier, *The Wall Street Journal*, in a reporting coup literally worthy of Hollywood, blew open the Theranos blood-testing scandal, which put the company's former top executive in jail.[42] All of these influential outlets have done significant coverage over the past decade on how the ACA is working—or not.

But with much greater attention in the media overall to who's up and who's down, this type of journalism has become harder to find and is restricted to a handful of outlets that most Americans don't read. In addition, national magazine coverage has declined, meaning those readers who want deep dives into health, public health, and science news have fewer places to go. Some magazines have shuttered; the once dominant *Time* and *Newsweek* are shadows of their former selves.

Moreover, when a health story starts to gain national traction, political reporters and health reporters clash over who gets to do a story, or the health reporter gets pushed aside—known in the trade as being "bigfooted." Health reporters don't want to go on the record sounding peevish about their colleagues, but this does happen at newspapers, TV and radio networks, and wire services. But behind the scenes, health reporters become frustrated when what started as a policy report morphs into today's gotcha political sound bite.

In these situations, it often works better for health reporters to partner with White House, congressional, or political reporters, to cover both the politics and policy in a way that is more nuanced and more accurate.

Amy Goldstein was a *Washington Post* reporter for more than three and a half decades. She covered a lot of beats, local and national, including the White House, and she wrote about lots of domestic policy, including an award-winning narrative nonfiction book about a Wisconsin town where the local General Motors plant shut down.[43]

But mostly she covered health, informing readers about policy and political dimensions of key issues. "I've written more about health care and health care policy than any other single thing I've written about," Goldstein told us about a year before joining several other experienced health reporters in taking a buyout when the *Post* sharply reduced its staff after missing financial goals. "But I like to think that no matter which beat I've had . . . I've really tried to write at the borderline. My attention is there between policy and politics because I think that they're really congruent."[44]

And even though she hadn't been a local reporter for decades, that experience early in her career instilled in her what she called "a sensibility about thinking how the federal government's decisions affect things at a local level, both politically at a local level, and consumers at a local level."[45] That ability to evoke the local story within the national story, illuminating the ground-level effects of federal decisions and political debates, has been a hallmark of her reporting.

And over the years, as health care has emerged as a top-tier political story, the *Post* has tended to team reporters up, rather than creating turf battles. A political, congressional, or White House reporter might team up with Goldstein or one of her colleagues on the health and science team. Or vice versa. "We'd collaborate," she said, particularly on the "what does this policy mean" part of the story.[46]

Cultural Bias in the Newsroom

Within newsrooms, the culture favors political reporting as the driving force and the political (and White House) beats as high status. A policy reporter might cover a health issue for months, but when a bill reaches the Senate floor or becomes a focus of White House messaging, a political, White House, or senior congressional reporter may step in without having a grasp of the nuances, the history, or the technicalities—and this occurs at the state level too.

This "bigfooting"—as mentioned earlier—extends into television. Politics reporters are the ones in demand to fill airtime on horse-race-driven TV news and talk programs—so it's the same reporters who don't care as much about policy or at least don't know as much about policy who end up explaining policy on air. That includes the Sunday-morning public affairs shows, which are also now mostly devoted to political topics and political prognostication. That means that the journalists who do not cover and who rarely know all that much about mask mandates or Obamacare subsidies or overdose prevention strategies are the ones on TV explaining such issues.

When policy reporting does happen, it's often very negative, focusing far more on problems than solutions, potential or actual. It is extremely incremental—Senator So-and-So said this and Congresswoman What's-Her-Name said that. As press scholar and critic Jay Rosen says, this produces a form of incrementalist journalism in which stories are simultaneously overcovered and undercovered. A lot of words could be written or aired, without creating public understanding of an issue.[47] Rosen also notes that citizens have some responsibility too; becoming informed and sustaining democracy requires effort. (Yet as Benjamin Toff and his coauthors have noted in *Avoiding the News*, news avoidance is more common among groups that are already more politically disengaged and disadvantaged.)[48]

If the coverage depicts problems as unsolvable, that becomes self-fulfilling. Many stories about drug overdose, for example, never mention the availability of safe and effective treatments for substance use disorders. Gloom-and-doom policy reporting leads to negativity and pessimism and cynicism, which make solutions seem beyond reach. Without reporting on solutions or at least potential solutions, the media fuels a "sense of despair, that nothing can get better," said Besser of the Robert Wood Johnson Foundation, who has also led the CDC and been at ABC News.[49]

A movement to address this, aptly called Solutions Journalism (supported by the Robert Wood Johnson Foundation, among other philanthropies) has recently emerged. But too often in US papers, happy news stories about things that actually work or show promise of working, if covered at all, are fluff on the features page.

After two or three years of reporting extensively on all the Obamacare enrollment website fiascos, one of us, then the editor overseeing health coverage at *Politico*, suggested doing a story on how open enrollment season had finally started without any serious glitches. Her editor resisted, citing the newsroom cliché that planes landing safely aren't news. To his credit, the editor heard her out as she argued that this turnaround was newsworthy; after all, the "plane" had been flying for several years with its engines on fire and its wings falling off. They ran a substantive story. The frame was how President Barack Obama's administration had salvaged his signature domestic achievement, and that's a legitimate approach given the political attacks and turmoil. But along with that political focus, the coverage reported clearly on how the sign-up system was finally working for ordinary people, many of whom received federal subsidies or were eligible for Medicaid, who were shopping for and obtaining insurance, some for the first time in years.

The Struggle of an Expert Journalist

Even the rare exceptional TV journalist struggles in today's environment. TV health news skews toward medicine and consumer health, but when policy stories are aired, they aren't necessarily as closely tied to politics as in print media. Yet TV health reporting has other challenges. The segments are usually short, just a few minutes, and it's hard to tell a complicated, multipart policy story in that compressed amount of time. TV needs visuals. And sources have to be willing to go on the air. And when a story has a particular public health focus—and public health at its best is about preventing problems, rather than cleaning up after them—it's hard to illustrate something that was averted.

Celine Gounder is an infectious disease physician and public health expert who is now spending most of her time doing both podcasting and health journalism on network news. She loves her work, but she explained its inherent challenge. One example: trying to film a TV segment on extreme risk protection orders, or ERPOs—better known as red-flag laws. These orders try to keep guns out of the hands of people whom a court has deemed a danger to themselves or others.

"How do you get someone who has been issued an ERPO to go on camera and be interviewed about it?" Gounder asked. Yet without that, it's challenging to get such a story on the air. Similar barriers can arise, she said, in trying to tell stories about people in marginalized communities. Even when reporters and producers do find people who are willing to go on the air, those individuals may not be representative of the story the reporter is trying to shed light on.[50]

Anecdotes can make good stories, she said, because they can be outliers—surprising and out of the ordinary. But the outlier is not necessarily representative of the story the reporter is trying to tell. And if the subject matter is a "breakthrough," it may also be the case that the only people who can access the treatment have a lot more resources than most people, for whom it is out of reach. From a scientific perspective, it may be fascinating, Gounder said. "But it's not going to help most people, it's not going to apply to most people. So it has no impact at scale."[51] And there are other practical obstacles, such as the fact that the networks often want to film a segment in a place like New York or Washington—avoiding costly and time-consuming travel to another locale for an entire crew. But the setting can change how a story can be told or how it ends up being perceived.

Gounder added that many public health problems happen in places far from New York and Washington, but it's hard to cover them how and where she wants to cover them, even in her role at KFF Health News, which partners with CBS to produce her work. "In health journalism or medical journalism, so much of the country and so many kinds of issues are not covered." It's just not in the TV bloodstream, so to speak. "I think when COVID reporting subsided, a lot of anchors and reporters were like, Oh, thank God."[52]

The Limits of the "Verticals"

Some news organizations have attempted to fill the policy void. *Vox*, for instance, is dedicated to explanatory journalism, including significant coverage of health, science, and climate. But most of the new efforts to elevate policy news either put it a bit off to the side or are geared to a professional audience, with subscription price points that don't make them accessible to the general public. Not all of these initiatives have thrived, though some have done so well that they've spawned imitators. Health newsletters have proliferated, and some are available without a paid subscription. There are a couple of health policy podcasts too. But whether newsletters and podcasts are here to stay—or whether they will go the way of RSS feeds and blogs and vlogs—is not a sure thing. Some of the health newsletters have already disappeared, at least in their free incarnation. Another possible warning sign: When National Public Radio in early 2023 laid off 10 percent of its staff, it placed much of the blame on declining podcast revenue.[53] Of course, another breed of podcasts—like Joe Rogan's—emerged as powerful influences during the 2024 campaign, but while they may make news, they are not news gatherers or news outlets in the traditional sense, and they may spread false and misleading information as much as they inform.

The Washington Post's innovative *Wonkblog*, a path-making feature debuted in 2011 that dove deep into policy reporting and explanatory reporting, didn't survive more than a few years, first turning to more of an economic and business focus and then ceasing altogether by 2021. Later, the *Post* created a daily online newsletter, the *Health 202*, that synopsized significant health care news and does original reporting. It survived a round of newsletter cutting prompted by the *Post*'s budget pressures in late 2023 but it disappeared the following year, as the Post announced plans to develop a new suite of premium newsletters for business-focused subscribers.

The New York Times' Upshot, created a few years after *Wonkblog*, started with a heavy policy focus and remains the home of thoughtful reporters like Margot Sanger-Katz.

Like Goldstein, Sanger-Katz is drawn to stories where the politics and policy come together. "The policy questions are all about what is going to happen to people's lives. How are things going to work? Where is the dollar going to go? What are the downstream consequences of these ideas?" she said. "The politics is like, 'What is possible? What can be achieved?'"[54]

When policy and politics come together, "you can start to see—how could policy change? And what would be the effects of those changes? That's the stuff that's really interesting to me."[55]

Sanger-Katz occasionally contributes to a daily or breaking news story, but mostly she's deep in Upshot projects, which can take many weeks to complete. She works a lot with the graphics and data and interactive colleagues, to tell stories with both words and visuals. "I think the place where the Upshot can be most valuable is with these kinds of projects. Going deep on data, or a visualization, or just doing something a little bit weird and different from what my other colleagues would do."[56]

The Upshot still does that kind of deep policy coverage; nobody else does these types of projects with any such consistency. But the section isn't pure policy either; it's done its share of politics, particulary during campaign seasons. And the Upshot is not always featured prominently on the *Times* website or mobile app; the policy news may be excellent, but there are some days when the reader has to go to the policy news, rather than having the policy news come to the reader. The *Times* has a huge number of newsletters, but policy-focused ones are vastly outnumbered by newsletters on culture, entertainment, food, and sports. The only health-focused newsletter is *Well*, which is personal or consumer health more than policy.

Politico had a big health team, more than 20 reporters and editors at its peak, plus a few more on the staff of the smaller state offshoots who sometimes collaborated with the national team. The publication, which had started as purely focused on political news, became known for its health coverage. But getting a story onto prime real estate on the free *Politico* home page (instead of behind a paywall for subscribers) almost always required a prominent political or campaign angle. That didn't mean that there couldn't be a lot of good, strong policy news in such a story; there was. But it needed a political "hook" to get that coveted home page space. Most of the health news at *Politico*—

and it's similar at *Axios* and some other DC publications—is found in publications within publications called verticals. They offer sophisticated policy coverage, but most content is available only to subscribers, and subscriptions are costly. The intended audience is not the general reader but health care trade groups, big providers, lobbyists, legislatures, and some of the larger nonprofit organizations. Only a fraction of that news is reworked for the broader public, outside the paywall.

The verticals do good work. They have reporters who are on the beat full time or almost full time, and these journalists can acquire expertise and also serve as in-house resources for colleagues who may have to dip into a health story now and then. But these emerging forms of national journalism tend to be for the aficionados, the readers who have a particular professional interest, whether as a clinician, academic, public health professional, industry leader, or lobbyist. In the news buffet, the verticals are a side dish—tasty and nourishing, but not enough for a full meal. They keep a segment of the population well informed, and some of the work does find its way to front pages or viral social media posts. But by and large, the general public doesn't see much of this nuanced and detailed reporting. What the public sees is the horse race, the conflict, and often, the cynicism.

Defining the Media as the Enemy

A final unfortunate characteristic of today's national news environment is the demonization of reporters by Trump and other political leaders. Of course, politicians' tendency to attack and blame individual reporters or "the press" is nothing new. It's served Democrats and Republicans well as an applause line; newspapers and TV and reporters themselves make alluring bogeymen. Richard Nixon famously had reporters on his "enemies" list, and the hostility shaped White House–media relations thereafter. (Nixon once told Henry Kissinger, "Never forget, the press is the enemy, the press is the enemy. . . . Write that on the blackboard 100 times.")[57] Ronald Reagan didn't have that degree of hostility on a personal level, but his sobriquet "the Great

Communicator" recognized his mastery of going around the media and speaking directly to the public. Just about every other president, Democrat or Republican, had their own testy moments and attempted end runs.

But Donald Trump took antagonism against the establishment press to new heights—in ways that have undermined the ability of national reporters to develop trust and cover health.

In his first term, he openly attempted to undermine independent journalism, rebranding mainstream reporters as "Enemies of the People"—terminology that would have been familiar to anyone living under 20th-century dictatorships. Reporters covering politics had faced hostility at rallies and online abuse before Trump. But not violent undercurrents quite like this.[58] Folks who showed up at rallies wearing T-shirts that said "Rope. Tree. Journalist." weren't all that funny. Nor were they intended to be. Trump had turned the Fourth Estate into the fifth column.

Shunning traditional networks, first as a candidate and then as president, Trump relied on Twitter, where he could say whatever he wanted, and Fox, a friendly platform with its arms wide open to him. He called for investigating journalists and their sources, floated the prosecution of journalists critical of him, and threatened to upend libel laws.[59] His administration memorably yanked the White House press credentials of a CNN reporter who asked tough questions.[60] Trump told his followers that it was all "fake news"—and that would come to include any health and science news that didn't fit into his preferred narrative.

The attacks and belittlement bore fruit. In a Hill-Harris survey released in July 2019—before the coronavirus emerged and before the 2020 campaign got underway—pollsters asked, "Which comes closer to your point of view: The news media is the enemy of the people, or the news media is an important part of democracy?" Fifty-one percent of Republican respondents chose the first option.[61] Asked about his attacks on "fake news," Trump told CBS's Lesley Stahl in 2016, "I do it to discredit you all, and demean you all, so that when you write negative stories about me, no one will believe you."⁶² It was perhaps one of the most candid, and prophetic, statements of his presidency.

In his second term, in its early months as we write this, Trump's relationship with the press has deteriorated even further. The White House has defied all sorts of precedents, including setting new rules about who can have access to or travel with the president, and favoring new conservative outlets. This antagonistic relationship has not at this point been focused specifically on health coverage; the first rounds have been focused on politics and defense. But concern is high that health reporters will have little access to policymakers at the White House, the Department of Health and Human Services, and its component health agencies, as programs get cut or revamped and Washington eyes historic changes to entitlements, social welfare programs, disease surveillance, and public health.

The erosion of trust in media has consequences far beyond coverage of one divisive president. According to Gallup, Americans' trust in the media, on the decline for years, particularly among Republicans and independents, nose-dived in 2020, the first year of the pandemic. By then a majority of Republicans said they didn't trust the mass media to "report the news fully, accurately and fairly," and in that single year the distrust rose by 10 percentage points among Republicans.⁶³

This lack of confidence couldn't have come at a worse possible time. Low trust in media became an impediment to good public health communication and fueled the climate in which public health officials, ranging from the National Institutes of Health's Anthony Fauci to obscure local officers, were hounded and threatened for doing work aimed at saving lives.

During the COVID-19 pandemic, reputable news outlets, citing reputable scientists, reported that masks were a helpful protective measure. But Trump said the public health measures were part of a scheme to sabotage the economy and boost then-candidate Joe Biden. And that's what large swaths of the population heard. And health reporters covering the pandemic, and particularly vaccination, began to be vilified and threatened in the same way their political reporter colleagues had been during the campaign. In a disease outbreak that caused well over a million deaths, many preventable, the credibility of media too was a casualty.

And to complete a particularly vicious circle, the attacks on traditional media may be changing the American diet for news—turning people off from high-quality sources. In 2024, researchers at the University of Pennsylvania offered free subscriptions to state newspapers to 2,529 individuals. Just 44 subscribed. The authors concluded, "Contemporary local newspapers may face a demand-side dilemma: The engaged citizens who formerly read them now prefer national, partisan content."[64]

If the public sees the media establishment as the enemy—or if people come to expect news delivered in a partisan shell—Americans will seek out alternative sources that deliver. And these other sources are often a lot less reliable. Instead of reading an Associated Press story written by someone like Ricardo Alonso-Zaldivar, people will look to a Facebook post, a link forwarded from a friend, or a YouTube video. Those starting down this road can find themselves led by algorithms to more posts, links, and videos featuring an increasing number of falsehoods, lies, and conspiracy theories. In the next chapter, we'll explore the avalanche of misinformation and disinformation, and how the health and public health systems are trying to confront it.

• CHAPTER 3

The Flood of Misinformation

Brandy Zadrozny kept pictures of a dead nurse on a bulletin board in her bedroom.[1] Only the nurse wasn't really dead.

Zadrozny is an NBC correspondent, a pioneer covering the disinformation beat. She started reporting on disinformation more than a decade ago, focusing mostly on political extremism online. Her beat has also come to include the swamp of health conspiracies.

The "dead" nurse in question is named Tiffany Dover. In late 2020, as the COVID-19 vaccines were first rolling out, Dover was living in Alabama and working right across the Tennessee border at the Catholic Health Initiatives Memorial Hospital in Chattanooga. The hospital, known locally just as CHI Memorial, had selected Dover to be one of the first of its health care workers to get the shot. She had nursed seriously ill COVID-19 patients and was an attractive working mom in her early thirties with unusually bright blue eyes. The vaccination event, on December 17, 2020, would be streamed on social media and aired on local TV.

A few minutes after the needle went in, Dover was at the microphone, explaining how excited and relieved she and her fellow nurses were to get a shot that would protect them against a virus that was killing not just patients but some of their health care workers.

Then she passed out.

She recovered fast, returning to the microphone to explain that she has a minor health condition called overactive vagal response that makes her prone to fainting.[2] No big deal. Dover was used to it.

Big swaths of the internet, however, weren't interested in her quirky vagus nerve. Anti-vaxxers and conspiracy theorists—some halfway around the globe—decided that Dover was dead. Killed by the vaccine. Victim of the medical-industrial complex. And they concluded that her family and the hospital were part of an enormous cover-up to conceal the truth.[3]

Zadrozny was hooked on the story.[4] She wanted to understand how people could be so distrustful of the reporting of local and national news on vaccine safety that they fell deep into the conspiracy. She also wanted to prove them wrong. So she spent the next year on a cross-country odyssey to prove that Dover was alive—and to try to talk to her, face-to-face. She found scattered postvaccine snapshots of Dover on friends' and acquaintances' Facebook pages, depicting a family Christmas celebration, a kid's basketball game. She spotted Dover's Pinterest posts, in which the nurse mulled over home decor for her next house. She found a freshly signed mortgage document available in public records.

Zadrozny sat down and talked with anti-vaxxers and conspiracy theorists, showing them her painstakingly acquired documentation. But she couldn't dent their certainty that it was all a hoax, that a body double was posing as the very dead nurse. The reporter managed to make contact with some of Dover's relatives, but for the first year of her reporting, she never got a chance to talk to Dover herself, to see her with her own eyes. It appeared that Dover was still hoping that somehow the whole big mess that had uprooted her job, her life, her husband's life, her kids' lives, and the lives of her entire extended family would just go away if she waited it out and didn't make waves—or grant interviews.[5]

That radical disruption of normal life was part of why Zadrozny pursued the Dover story with such determination. "Because," she explained on the opening segment of the podcast series called *Tiffany Dover Is Dead*, "she represents what this larger phenomenon of misinformation is really about, a regular person whose life becomes a weapon in a global information war."[6]

"I didn't die that day," the nurse would eventually tell her, in an interview that finally took place after the initial five-part series aired, after Dover gave up hope that ignoring the people spinning the lies would make them just go away. "But the life I knew did."[7]

The Infodemic

In one sense, misinformation and disinformation are as old as humanity itself. Just ask Adam and Eve and that snake. People have always made mistakes, and they have always lied. In public health, there's a long history of falsehoods that have cost lives.

Think of the "snake oil peddlers" with their patents and potions a century or so ago. The tobacco executives who claimed smoking doesn't really cause lung cancer. The conspiracy theorists who think abortion causes breast cancer.[8] The powerful congressional committee chairman who, after 9/11 and the anthrax letter attacks, quizzed heads of US military bioresearch labs about why they were spending so much of their time and effort and federal dollars developing an anthrax vaccine rather than a homeopathic cure.[9] And of course those misinforming about vaccination, who have been at it since the first doses of the smallpox vaccine were administered centuries ago.

What makes falsehoods so compelling? Many researchers who study communication and misinformation argue that humans are hardwired to believe information they encounter, at least initially. As RTI health communications scholar Brian Southwell and his colleagues have pointed out, that assertion of our default trust dates back to at least Spinoza.[10]

But now, in the digital age, misinformation and disinformation spread at a scale and speed unprecedented in history. People find misinformation—or it finds them. They also find other people, huge numbers of other people, who believe in it, reinforcing false beliefs and creating an instant community. A study published in *Science* tracked stories that had been retweeted millions of times on Twitter—and this was Twitter 1.0, before Elon Musk.[11] The researchers found that items that were unequivocally false traveled "farther, faster, deeper, and more broadly" than accurate ones. The top 1 percent of stories reached between 1,000 and 100,000 people, "while true statements rarely diffused to more than 1,000."[12] And it was people, not bots, doing the spreading.

The goal of disinformation is more than to sow confusion about facts. Its aim is to confuse, to undermine, to erode, and to divide. And, sometimes, to make money. Health and science are a casualty. So are social cohesion and trust. People may find instant communities online, but nowadays, in our fractured society, as misinformation expert Renée DiResta pointed out in *Invisible Rulers: The People Who Turn Lies into Reality*, being part of one community often puts us on the other side of an uncrossable line from other communities.[13]

The more novel the disinformation, the more it elicits outrage, fear, hostility, or other negative emotions and the faster it flies. That intense engagement may boost the social media platforms' bottom line. But it has had a profound and damaging impact on the health of individuals and of communities. It is entwined with distrust of the US health care system and the scientific enterprise in general, including in marginalized communities.

The general and prolonged anxiety of the pandemic era and its aftermath—economic, social, and medical—only made people more receptive to misinformation and conspiracy theories. It is not hyperbole to say that disinformation kills. The vaccine didn't kill Tiffany Dover. But misinformation about the vaccine contributed to the deaths of people who believed until it was too late that the vaccine is more lethal than the virus.[14]

It has also harmed, or killed, people who shun other vaccines or proven treatments in favor of baseless fads or "alternative" remedies.

Misinformation is now everywhere. TV. Radio. Print. Email chains. WhatsApp groups. Political campaigns. The office water cooler. The gym locker room. The family Thanksgiving table. And of course social media. We are all exposed to it, again and again and again. And we've all lived through what the World Health Organization has called an "infodemic"—the spread of "false or misleading information in digital and physical environments during a disease outbreak." An infodemic, WHO says, "causes confusion and risk-taking behaviors that can harm health. It also leads to mistrust in health authorities and undermines the public health response."[15]

One reason it's been easy for people in a divided society to believe that their government is lying to them is the fact that governments do—sometimes—lie, spin, and misinform. Vietnam, Watergate, and the assertions about weapons of mass destruction in Iraq loom large in national memory banks; other governments have lied about everything from their own national debt to the coronavirus toll or why they've begun a war. As Sophia Rosenfeld, a historian at the University of Pennsylvania, noted in her book *Democracy and Truth: A Short History*, truth can exist without democracy; biologists and engineers and the like can and do advance knowledge under a dictatorship or authoritarian regime. But democracy is different. Democracy "cannot survive without any commitment to verifiable truth and truth telling from either the population at large or the powers on high."[16]

But the broad trust that requires is threatened today. There's a difference between healthy skepticism about government and a wholesale disregard for any and all government information. Nor is distrust aimed solely at government. It's aimed at scientists. At doctors and nurses. At the health system. At public health workers. At journalists. And at one another.

Much of the misinformation and disinformation involve our health. A study published in the *Journal of Cancer Education* back in 2018—well before the upheaval of the coronavirus—found that nearly one in three social media articles about cancer contained misinformation. Three-fourths of that misinformation was harmful, in the sense that the information could send patients away from, not toward, the best treatments and therapies. Another worrisome finding was that people stayed engaged online with the erroneous content longer than with the accurate content.[17] Those engagement patterns are common with "fake news" and disinformation. "Real" news gets an online spike and then people move on. Fake news, misinformation, and conspiracy theories not only engage people longer but diffuse over time, with tropes re-emerging again and again, often in more radical form.[18]

As if the problem weren't already bad enough, artificial intelligence is threatening to make it worse. NewsGuard, an organization founded by journalist Steven Brill to address misinformation, is tracking AI-generated sites that are "operating with little to no human oversight"—and has found many hundreds.[19] According to NewsGuard, the sites obtain revenue through advertising, incentivizing the creation of content that draws readers. "Some of these sites are generating hundreds if not thousands of articles a day," one researcher at NewsGuard told *The Washington Post*. "This is why we call it the next great misinformation superspreader."[20]

There is also rising concern about the use of AI to generate deepfakes to deceive about elections, climate, and health.[21] Of course, AI is evolving so rapidly that predicting exactly how and how much it will propel disinformation is not possible. It's also important to remember that AI is not only in the hands of the fake-news-producing villains; so far, it's widely accessible to all. So if AI surpasses humans in its ability to *produce* disinformation, it could also surpass humans in its ability to *detect* disinformation. Darren Linvill, codirector of the Media Forensics Hub at Clemson University, suggests the future may lie somewhere in between the extremes—a revved-up, more automated version of the information wars that have gone on for decades. "It's still the same fundamental tension," Linvill said. "Bad guys are going to use computers to do their job. . . . Good guys are going to use computers to try to counter the bad guys."[22]

Defining the Terms

"Misinformation" is commonly defined as information that is incorrect or false in the context of scientific understanding of the times. It is often the result of ignorance or poor understanding—and well-intentioned reporters can be guilty of it when, as we saw in earlier chapters, they don't have the time, resources, mentoring, or training to get things right.

Disinformation is purposefully created and disseminated falsehoods.

One is error. The other is lies.

That distinction was made at least as far back as the 1980s.[23] Not all experts accept these definitions, however, or think they continue to be useful in today's context. When something begins as an honest mistake—misinformation—but gets repeated, amplified, and deliberately touted ad infinitum, at some point it morphs into disinformation, and there's no way to precisely identify that line.

Honest errors can also become weaponized as disinformation. But it may not matter whether it's *dis-* or *mis*information so much as who is spreading it and why. Someone who randomly shares on social media a bit of misinformation that he or she found interesting is different from someone who is sharing it because they have political or economic motives to undermine public health authorities, discredit vaccines, or peddle their own "natural" products instead.

The Center for Countering Digital Hate dubbed the 12 most prolific anti-vax voices of social media, including Robert F. Kennedy Jr. before he became HHS Secretary, the "Disinformation Dozen."[24] Their sites were generally selling products along with their ideology; the center estimated that the anti-vax industry brings in at least $36 million a year.[25] Many of these prominent voices in health disinformation are also conspiracy theorists, meaning they have "specific characteristics, such as the belief that a hidden group of powerful individuals exerts control over some aspect of society."[26]

And some are propagandists—meaning that the information they peddle, some of which might be true, is designed to "disparage opposing viewpoints" and win people over to a political group or party.[27]

Some of the disinformation is not made in America, but manufactured by foreign actors. The 2022 report *Memes, Magnets and Microchips*, by the Stanford Internet Observatory's Virality Project, distinguished between homegrown and imported misinformation, identifying Russia, China, and Iran as the lead global players.[28]

Disinformation and Equity

While disinformation is pervasive and targets pretty much everyone, some disinformation campaigns aim at specific racial or ethnic populations, including Black Americans and Hispanic Americans. These groups may already have a higher baseline of distrust in the US health care and public health systems, based on both historical and contemporary mistreatment. And they tend to have "poorer information ecosystems and impoverished access to high-quality information" compared with more affluent and predominantly white communities, prompting Sara Gorman to argue that it is "increasingly appropriate to view information environments as a social determinant of health."[29] Some of the race- or ethnic-focused narratives don't start out aimed at a specific population but evolve that way as they travel through these communities.

Others grow "organically" in minority communities, as researchers at First Draft put it.[30] "Vaccine shedding and its alleged effects on women's reproductive health is a narrative that started in white anti-vaccine spaces and was amplified to Black online communities by Black anti-vaccine influencers," they wrote in 2021. "On the other hand, vaccine classism and the idea that Black people would receive an inferior vaccine is a narrative that our research shows originated in Black online conversations." They added that certain narratives that circulate broadly, such as the idea that the COVID-19 vaccines were "experimental, rushed and unsafe," can become "much more intricate and multi-layered" given that, historically, experiments were conducted on Black people. The fertility memes resonate in minority communities, too, because of the history of forced sterilization. In chapter 5, we'll see how some new nonprofit news outlets are arising for and within neglected and minority communities, which may fortify efforts to rebuild trust in news and health information. This dynamic is something that academics, clinicians, and public health officials should be cognizant of as they attempt to counter and get ahead of misinformation, as discussed in chapter 6.

Academic Challenges

Misinformation is especially challenging in the academic world, which values the freedom for faculty to consider unconventional ideas. When a single professor makes a false accusation or posts unreliable information, misinformation peddlers are quick to associate it with their institution, either through identification of the author or through an assertion that it represents an institution-backed study.

This challenge is personified by Scott Atlas, a Stanford University radiologist—not an infectious disease expert or epidemiologist—who had left the medical school in 2012. He had pivoted to health policy at the Stanford-affiliated Hoover Institution. (He later maintained that health policy experts, not epidemiologists or virologists, should be front and center in the pandemic.)[31] Early in the pandemic, Atlas appeared multiple times on Fox News, where he was identified as a Stanford doctor, an affiliation that bestowed credibility and prestige. Atlas put out information that downplayed the danger of COVID-19 and called for a "herd immunity" strategy. The faculty senate at Stanford later overwhelmingly voted to condemn his role in spreading damaging messaging during the pandemic.[32] Nonetheless, his words were broadly disseminated, confusing the public. He later clashed with public health officials as a White House adviser to President Donald Trump.[33]

Differential Susceptibility

People handle misinformation in different ways. Some read it, process it, and reject it. Some are confused or uncertain—but potentially persuadable, perhaps by a physician or a nurse or a community health worker or some other trusted person or source of information. Others go deep, deep, deep down the rabbit hole—and stay there.

Misinformation is "sticky." That means it's hard to change the minds of those who are very dug in, particularly those who may not come into contact with doctors or nurses or other health workers very often and who aren't particularly trustful of them when they do. About 40 percent of Americans did not have a single encounter with a primary care provider, let alone an ongoing relationship, in a year, according to one oft-cited study.[34] Some of them are young and healthy and just don't see a need for a doctor, or they worry about the cost of care. But a subset of Americans have lost faith in medicine, or the medical establishment. And that population is ripe for disinformation. These are people who would still insist Nurse Dover is dead even if they were standing right next to her in the checkout line at their local grocery store.

Another set of people who have been exposed to misinformation are hesitant or uncertain but not intractably opposed to traditional science-based medicine or public health measures, whether it's cancer treatment or immunization. It's this middle group, people who have doubts or fears or questions—which can be both reasonable and understandable—but who haven't slammed doors shut, that is, for now, the richer target for credible, accurate messaging. This is particularly true if they are still "patients," if they have some connection to and trust in their doctor, nurse, or other care provider. This is why it's important that clinicians—not just doctors, nurses, and physician's assistants but everyone who comes into contact with patients—learn some basics about answering patient questions and calming their fears. (For more on the role of clinicians and resources for them, see chapter 6.)

During the COVID-19 vaccination drive, for instance, the share of the population that were "never" or "anti" vaxxers didn't budge very much. Indeed, it rose a little bit as vaccination got more highly politicized on the right. According to the KFF COVID-19 Vaccine Monitor (also supported by the Robert Wood Johnson Foundation), which conducted nearly monthly surveys, 15 percent of adults said they would "never" get the COVID-19 shot in December 2020 when the vaccines were rolling out. By April 2022, after more than a year of having the vaccine free and readily available, it was roughly the same—17 percent.

In contrast, in December 2020, 39 percent said they'd "wait and see" about getting immunized. Then the outreach and education (and to some extent the mandates) worked on this group—the uncertain middle. By April 2022, only 4 percent said they'd "wait and see." Most Americans had gotten at least one dose of the vaccine.[35]

This doesn't mean that the public health and health care worlds should write off the people who are most dug in and hostile. It does mean that, for now, the limited collective wisdom we have on fighting misinformation will be most effective on the "persuadable." Even with that goal in mind, fundamental questions remain about how to identify and promote the most credible messengers and the most credible messages. It's still far from clear how the truth tellers will be able to keep up with, let alone outrun, the deniers of truth.

The Toolbox for Countering Misinformation

Today's infodemic is not a secret. As our colleagues at the Johns Hopkins Center for Health Security wrote, a partial list of concerned global and national agencies includes "international/intergovernmental organizations (WHO, UNICEF, UNICRI, UNESCO, UNAOC, PAHO, EU, ESCTF, and the European Commission); US federal government agencies and programs (HRSA, FBI, Office of the US Surgeon General, CISA, CDC, FEMA, DHS, AARP, FDA, HHS, DOJ, the White House, USAID, US Marine Corps, and the Global Engagement Center)." It's no acronym left behind.[36]

Unfortunately, rising interest in the problem has not been matched by the development of effective solutions. To be sure, there are now more tools to counter disinformation than existed a few years ago. Unfortunately, none of these tools has proved to be a silver bullet. They may help some of the people some of the time, but the scale of misinformation and disinformation remains overwhelming.

As a result, some experts are advocating for the implementation of multiple tools to counter misinformation simultaneously. Similar to how public health officials talk about a "Swiss cheese" approach to a virus or other outbreak, meaning layering one good but imperfect defense on another until all the holes are covered, misinformation experts see promise in hitting the problem from different sides at once. At least for now, this may be the best chance to help more of the people more of the time, as society struggles to find more systematic ways to protect itself.

Let's turn to exploring today's toolbox, which includes fact checking, debunking, inoculating and prebunking, surveillance and monitoring, rapid responses, strengthening credible sources, and mobilizing in real life.

Fact Checking

It seems so simple. If wrong information is out there, just correct it! Unfortunately it's anything but simple, and fact checking, though essential, may be limited in its reach. Awash in both misinformation and factual information, people have trouble figuring out which is which. And as we've noted, once a mistaken belief, or worse, a conspiracy theory, takes hold in someone's mind or worldview, it sticks, making it hard to dislodge.

Many people never see fact checking. Others have drunk so deeply from conspiratorial wells that they wouldn't believe it if they did see it. That doesn't mean fact checking and debunking are useless. They do provide some degree of accountability and, coming from reliable, trustworthy sources, they can help people—that persuadable middle—who do want to discern fact from fiction in the world of information overload we all inhabit. Of note, a few studies have found that people have more confidence in journalists confirming something is true than reporting that something is wrong.[37]

Fact checking—holding people accountable for what they say, write, or post—remains a core function of journalism in any democracy. In recent years, as information has spread and morphed further and faster on multiplying platforms and channels, fact checking has become a subgenre of journalism. It can take several forms. Sometimes it unfolds close to real time, as when news organizations check statements politicians are making in a debate, rally, or similar event. President Trump's daily coronavirus press conferences during the first year of the pandemic got a lot of rapid scrutiny as he veered away from the best available science or minimized the pandemic threat. His musing about ingesting bleach to kill the coronavirus was the most notorious example, but reporters highlighted dozens of less bizarre but still damaging assertions.

Beyond these instant checks, many national outlets do deeper "fact check" accountability articles to clear up confusion, misstatements, or distortions in a more detailed and systematic way. These aren't immediate but they are fast—fast enough that the comments and assertions in question are still fresh. Often they delve into political claims—a statement that an elected official or candidate made in a speech, debate, or news conference, whether the error or exaggeration was inadvertent or intentional.

Health and science claims get fact-checked too. This was common during the pandemic, the mpox outbreak, and other fast-moving health stories. And fact-checkers combat false claims about other issues ranging from climate change (which is also a public health issue) to crime to immigration. They often home in on statistics that have been mangled or misused, whether intentionally or inadvertently. Various media watch groups on the left and right also do versions of fact checking, though not necessarily in real time and sometimes with a more partisan perspective.

News organizations also have fact-check features. *The Washington Post*, for instance, does fairly detailed analysis not just of politicians' statements and misstatements but of policy claims, health and otherwise. It awards untrue statements up to four "Pinocchios"—although the paper added a "Bottomless Pinocchio" for President Trump in his first term—and Joe Biden subsequently earned a few of his own, too.[38]

During the pandemic, the fact-check feature was quite focused on vaccination, the Chinese "lab leak" controversy, and false attacks on then–National Institute of Allergy and Infectious Diseases director Anthony Fauci. It called Senator Ron Johnson, a Wisconsin Republican, a one-man disinformation campaign "undeterred by fact checkers, federal health agencies, medical experts and a growing body of scientific research."[39]

In response to the inundation of misinformation, the Associated Press created a dedicated fact-checking team, too. Some of their articles get distributed on the Associated Press wire like any other story, but most are linked to websites with a tag. In other words, if someone is doing a Google search on something that may be contentious or distorted online, a little notification beneath it tells the searcher that a fact-check is available. At times social media platforms have added similar tags to controversial content.

The Associated Press assembled a team of reporters to specialize in dismantling myths and explaining the underlying truth. For instance, when a test became available that could check someone for both flu and COVID-19, misinformation circulated that this "proved" that COVID-19 and the flu were the same disease. The Associated Press fact-check explained it did not.[40]

"What we do a lot of is just looking essentially online to see what people are talking about," said journalist Graph Massara, who worked on that Associated Press team for a time and who spent months "training" his own TikTok algorithms to serve up the bad stuff so he could track and try to counter it.[41] That means monitoring the gamut of social media platforms: Twitter, Facebook, Instagram, Google platforms, and so forth. And they have to be claims that the Associated Press can truly take apart.

"A lot of this job is figuring out what is actually debunkable, meaning it's specific enough that we can *prove* it wrong," Massara said. "I can't sit here and be like 'UFOs have never happened, and the government is not lying to you about UFOs.' Because who am I going to confirm that with? The likelihood that I'm going to be able to definitively prove that as a negative is not good, so I can't debunk it."[42] However, he added, sometimes he could establish that a photo posted online of a "UFO" actually depicted a hot air balloon.

The fact-checkers also struggle when bad information comes from people who don't intend to deceive. They may have just misunderstood something and posted it, and then it took off.

"A lot of these most persistent rumors come from a study or a survey, or something that somebody at some point misunderstood," Massara said. But he noted that when he reached out to scientists to help smash these rumors, they often responded with caution and a boatload of caveats. That's necessary in the world of research and academia but doesn't pack enough punch for ordinary people. That reluctance to speak in absolutes, to come out and say explicitly that something is wrong, is a challenge to fact-checkers, who necessarily have to communicate in a pretty straightforward way to people seeking certitude. "It's not helpful because something can be 98 percent wrong and they're not going to say it's wrong because that's how science works," said Massara. "But most people don't understand how science works."[43]

In addition to media outlets' fact checking, there are a few excellent online fact-checking sites, the best known being FactCheck.org and PolitiFact. (We include some fact-checking resources for the general public in chapter 7, "Protecting Yourself—and Others.")

A project of the Annenberg Public Policy Center of the University of Pennsylvania, FactCheck.org was established in 2003 to check politicians' veracity, which can include claims about health care cost and coverage and about public health. Later, the site added a SciCheck section, which examines statements about everything from autism to climate to mammograms. It also added "Viral Spiral," a feature that helps people detect bogus stories and "fake news."

Originally, the site was designed to help people figure out how much—if any—truth there was in the then-ubiquitous email chain letters, a leading vessel for misinformation before social media displaced it with far broader amplification. The fact-checking resources have let readers find out that the Biden administration wasn't handing out "crack pipes" to facilitate drug use; it was funding harm reduction programs proven to reduce the spread of disease. That Fauci did not subject caged beagles to sand fly bites as part of an experiment. That Trump didn't tell *People* magazine in 1998 that if he ever made a run for the White House, he'd run as a Republican because "they're the dumbest group of voters in the country."[44]

The site takes readers' questions, and it also has a search function so people can check out what they hear, about politics or health, whether it's on social media or in their in-laws' kitchen. For obvious reasons, a lot of the health focus has been on vaccination. FactCheck.org got out very early on the misinformation about RSV vaccines that was bubbling up even before the first shot was administered.[45] It posted several articles about measles as the outbreak spread in the winter of 2025.[46] It has also increasingly focused on false assertions about climate change.

PolitiFact, run by the Poynter Institute, is a similar site. It too is politics focused but also has addressed COVID-19, health care, marijuana, and gay rights. It ranks statements on a six-point "Truthometer," running from True and Mostly True to "Pants on Fire." In addition to holding politicians accountable, it takes down some of the false information on social media. One example, which PolitiFact termed a "zombie claim" because it keeps recirculating, is a photo purporting to be a dead Hillary Clinton lying on a "lethal medical injection" table.[47]

Poynter also launched the International Fact-Checking Network in 2015 to train and connect fact-checkers around the globe. That in turn led to the #CoronaVirusFacts alliance, started in January 2020 and available in more than 40 languages.[48] At the time, Poynter noted, the virus hadn't yet spread beyond China (at least, it hadn't been detected outside China), but the misinformation was already rampant across the globe.

Factchequeado, jointly initiated by the Spanish nonprofit Maldita.es and the Argentina-based Chequeado, counters misinformation for the 60 million people within the US Hispanic and Latino communities.[49] Those communities rely heavily on social media for news, including WhatsApp. Factchequeado is available on a variety of platforms and social networks, plus it collaborates and does training with other Latino media and fact-checking organizations, including the main Spanish-language television networks seen in the United States. Its crowdsourcing components help it address the different Hispanic and Latino communities across the country.

The organization started with more of a political focus; it wasn't created in response to the pandemic per se, said cofounder Laura Zommer in a WhatsApp interview from Argentina. But as it began to address the virus and vaccination misinformation, it became clear that there were some basic underlying disinformation types that crossed subject matter—politics, health, whatever. And that the disinformation ricocheted around the world. "What the Coronavirus made absolutely evident for all the world is that there were narratives that were global—and that the approach for this information should be at the same time global and hyperlocal," Zommer said. (She also recalled the irony of covering some politicians who were bashing lifesaving vaccines in rich countries while politicians in poor countries were desperately trying to get supplies of the expensive shots for their own people.)[50]

Public health is not Factchequeado's sole domain; voting and immigration are also priority topics. But public health and vaccination are key. In addition to helping train journalists who serve Spanish-speaking communities in the United States, the organizations has been training pediatricians and other health workers on the front lines.

But if fact checking thrives on the national, or even international, stage, it is sparse on the local level. Governors, mayors, state lawmakers, and other local officials don't have to worry much about someone looking over their untruthful shoulder, according to research from the Duke Reporters' Lab at the Sanford School of Public Policy.[51]

This gap in accountability often plays out in the news deserts described in earlier chapters. As of 2023, at least 25 states did not have a state or local media outlet that fact-checked politicians on a regular basis. (Poynter's PolitiFact does have some state editions, but they are limited.) "The smaller the office, the less likely was scrutiny," the Duke team reported. "Out of 7,386 state legislative seats, just 47 of those lawmakers were checked (0.6%)," it said. "And among the more than 1,400 U.S. mayors of cities of 30,000 people or more, just seven were checked. (0.5%)."[52]

That means that candidates or officials propagating falsehoods about climate change or drugs or vaccines or masks or homelessness or gun safety go unchallenged. Even if a political opponent does call out the falsehoods, it can be hard for ordinary people to know truth from untruth if there isn't some kind of neutral, reliable fact checking to step in. Is candidate A lying? Or is candidate B? People often vote based on their loyalty to a political party, not on who is telling them the truth. Sometimes they vote for their political party even if they know the candidate isn't telling the truth.[53]

Machine learning and artificial intelligence, which are evolving rapidly, have the potential to add to fact checking. Google and other tech firms are already deploying machine learning to detect images that have been manipulated as well as deep fakes. In theory, AI tools might be able to spot assertions that are not true. The Duke Reporters' Lab—which includes the journalist who founded PolitiFact—has developed a prototype for a fact-check that would pop up on a TV screen during a presidential news conference or debate. The lab playfully named it Squash—"chosen because it is a nutritious vegetable and a good metaphor for stopping falsehoods."[54] Sadly, the rise of AI-based fact checking raises the specter of an arms race between the AI spewing misinformation and the AI trying to stop it.

Debunking

Debunking aims to go beyond the basic "true-false" fact-check approach and address the larger cognitive context, including by exposing people to reliable online narratives. For instance, in one study, US Facebook users reduced their 2020 holiday season travel after they were shown ads where doctors and nurses warned about the dangers of COVID-19. The counties where such messages were shown saw reduced travel—and infection rates in those counties and zip codes decreased.[55]

In another international experiment, Facebook users exposed to information accurately depicting rising coronavirus vaccine acceptance were more likely to show more acceptance themselves.[56] Studies have also found benefits from having clinicians text video messages to their patients with COVID-19 information. Some found evidence that patients sought out more information when the health provider's race or ethnicity matched their own.[57] But overall, debunking's success remains limited. Sometimes it creates what's known as a backfire effect, causing people to double down in their false beliefs—although a recent wave of research indicates that backfiring is not as common and intractable as earlier scholarship suggested. And it's hard for debunkers to pierce myths and misinformation in an era when untold millions of people place more trust in "influencers" on social media or cable TV or widely followed podcasts than in legitimate, evidence-based medical and public health voices or the journalists who diligently try to disseminate their fact-based work and knowledge.

Even when debunking initially seems to work, its effect may be ephemeral. People revert to their previously held views, sometimes in as little as a week, according to research on misinformation from MIT political scientist Adam Berinsky.[58] He and others have identified an additional conundrum with debunking: If a rumor is debunked once, it has limited impact because it just doesn't change that many minds for that long. But if it's debunked repeatedly, it gains "fluency"—meaning the rumor travels more easily. That is where backfiring may come into play. One debunking doesn't make an impression. But, perversely, repeated debunkings may reinforce the incorrect belief.

Debunking, fact checking, and even credible messengers can't force people to engage with the truth. Even a decade ago, before misinformation became an infodemic, researchers looked at 50,000 debunking posts on Facebook from 2010–2014 and found engagement was suboptimal.[59]

"Fact-checking and correction efforts hinge on the assumption that people engage with information in an objective, rational way," another set of scholars wrote later, focusing on the pandemic. But if everyone were engaging with information in an objective, rational way, we wouldn't have a disinformation crisis. Instead, multiple factors, including cognitive biases, distrust in expertise, and emotions like fear and anxiety, can undermine our efforts to unwind misinformation.[60] How to delink those anxieties from a receptiveness toward disinformation is not yet well understood.

Inoculation

Other tools in the anti-misinformation toolbox are inoculation and the related concept of prebunking. Sometimes these terms are used interchangeably, but it's useful to think about inoculation as building defenses against misinformation in general and prebunking as an attempt to get ahead of a specific pernicious claim or campaign. Both are preventive, sharing the basic goal of helping people recognize and resist disinformation before it does its harm.

Inoculation involves teaching people, via online platforms or free online games developed for this purpose, about the manipulative techniques of disinformation. That recognition helps them detect it and resist it. It's called inoculation because the exposure is modeled on how a vaccine trains the immune system to recognize and fight back against disease. Inoculation often relies on games like *Bad News*, created (reportedly, and suitably, in a bar) by the Cambridge Social Decision-Making Lab with DROG, a Dutch media collective, and graphic design agency Gusman.[61] *Bad News* shows players how to gain followers and credibility by playing on emotions—including outrage and anxiety—to build a malevolent online "fake news" presence.

In 2020, the University of Cambridge, the UK Cabinet Office, and WHO released *Go Viral!*, another free online game in which players learn to manipulate claims to stir up outrage. The Cambridge team is also behind *Harmony Square*, where a player is the chief disinformation officer who destroys a community's harmony. The Cambridge researchers who developed these games, notably Jon Roozenbeek and Sander van der Linden, have found they create a kind of intellectual armament, as though a red-alert system had been installed in people's brains so that when they encounter misinformation they recognize it.

The idea is that acquired "mental antibodies" can detect and resist what van der Linden describes as the six key tools of disinformation—discrediting/denial/deflection, emotional appeals, polarization, conspiracy theories, trolling, and impersonation of experts.[62] One strength of the approach is that the Cambridge researchers have found it works across different cultures. Outside the public health sphere, inoculation models have also been used to combat right-wing radicalization and white supremacy among US youth, particularly through an American University program called the Polarization and Extremism Research and Innovation Lab.[63] First Draft News also developed some simple online classes to help people learn to spot falsehoods and to use tools and techniques like geolocation to verify information.[64]

Prebunking can be specific, an attempt to get ahead of a certain strain of misinformation that is detected or anticipated. It often uses social media sites like YouTube and TikTok to build these fortresses of fact. Prebunking can also focus on foundational themes and narratives rather than a specific claim, tackling "the broader persistent narratives of misinformation beyond specific claims."[65] It can educate people about conspiracy theories in general. Prebunking can involve texts, graphics, and videos. But while it's relatively easy to do a simple fact-based prebunking campaign, it's not clear that it has much lasting impact. The "mental antibodies" of games seem to stick in people's minds longer than these specific campaigns.[66]

As disinformation research expands, it's reasonable to expect that it will come up with more refined techniques that yield a more enduring response.

Prebunking also faces practical barriers in getting into the online platforms where it's most needed. It's easy to post a debunking video on YouTube. It's a lot harder to gain entry to and disseminate prebunking messages to the target audience in closed systems like WhatsApp or Telegram. (One Factchequeado initiative includes a WhatsApp chat bot, where people can submit statements, videos, or images to get them fact-checked.)[67] Nor have there yet been, to our knowledge, successful efforts to get public health messaging or prebunking themes into pop culture, the way HIV storylines were part of television 20 years ago, when HIV was misunderstood and stigmatized.

It's also hard to figure out what specifically needs to be prebunked—and the window is narrow. Some false campaigns can be anticipated; warnings about autism, infertility, and the like were straight out of the anti-vax playbook. And some of the playbook is familiar. As the Stanford Internet Observatory's *Memes, Magnets and Microchips* report said, the playbook has four main categories—lack of safety, distribution (such as the claim that vaccines exist primarily to make profits for the drug industry), efficacy, and conspiracy.[68]

But a fundamental challenge with inoculation and prebunking is that it's hard to predict the wild claims that circulate above and beyond that familiar playbook. Would anyone have dreamed up a prebunking campaign for the COVID-19 shots around the idea that Bill Gates was implanting microchips in our bodies? Or that vaccines contain the eggs of a tentacled parasite? By early 2023, a video making that assertion had been viewed more than a million times.[69]

Prebunking these kinds of messages requires both an early general bulwark against the overarching themes and a kind of real-time hotspotting of the specifics. Groups doing this work need to develop far greater speed and agility, and their messages need to have staying power. Failure to defeat coronavirus vaccine disinformation spurred greater opposition to routine childhood vaccines, despite their long-established records of efficacy and safety and broad acceptance. And that has further empowered critics of the vaccines to try to weaken state requirements for school-age children.

Surveillance and Rapid Response

Some successful campaigns provide hope for fighting against misinformation. Working closely with community-based organizations, New York City's Department of Health and Mental Hygiene, for instance, opened an ambitious misinformation surveillance program during the early phase of COVID-19 vaccination. They watched (and listened to) what was bubbling up or being amplified on social media, in neighborhood leaflets, and on other channels in various communities, including among Black residents, Orthodox Jews, and Russian and Latin American immigrants, as well as political conservatives, and then tried to counter the messages.[70]

The city's response was initially led by a group known as the Misinformation Team, a name that was later changed to the Community Concerns Team. While all this was going on, the city's health commissioner at the time, Dave Chokshi, managed to spend at least two days a month taking care of patients at a Bellevue clinic for unhoused patients. That firsthand contact helped him understand what people were seeing, hearing—and fearing. He was able to loop that real-life feedback back into the city's messaging.[71]

More recently, a group based out of Washington University in St. Louis's Brown School of Public Health has set up information and disinformation monitoring in about a dozen cities, mostly in the Midwest, with weekly reports about what people in the community are hearing. It's small scale, but it does give public health officials a fairly quick window on what's out there—and they've found considerable community conversation about mental health, not just respiratory viruses, said Matthew Kreuter, an expert on public health communications at the Brown School, who has helped develop iHeard St. Louis and who is part of the team taking the approach into other communities.[72]

Several dozen health organizations, ranging from small nonprofits to big foundations and from large health systems to pharmaceutical companies, have formed the Coalition in Health and Science to try to promote fact-based health information and to become a rapid-response force. The goal is to detect the disinformation and share it with member organizations, facilitating a rapid response to head off or dispel it. "If something emerges tomorrow . . . every single communication person in every one of those 50 organizations will send that correct information through the ecosystem the same day," said Reed Tuckson, a prime organizer of the coalition.[73]

In another effort, the Public Good Projects (PGP) are doing a big sweep of multiple online sources, reporting to public health officials, researchers, and clinicians. They put together a monthly email report. But the monthly cadence, while quite helpful for clinicians and frontline health workers dealing with uncertain or nervous patients, is more useful for debunking campaigns than for prebunking. Once lies have been around a month, they've planted roots. PGP has teamed up with a consortium of other public health organizations to disseminate key information more quickly.[74] KFF, formerly known as the Kaiser Family Foundation (and the parent of KFF Health News, discussed in the next chapter), has also begun a major disinformation initiative, monitoring emerging online trends and sharing updates twice a month at no charge with public health practitioners and researchers, journalists, and the general public.[75]

Strengthening Credible Sources

Disinformation researchers have noted that the right "credible communicator"—often an unexpected one—can sometimes break through. It's inconsistent though. For instance, a conservative Georgia Republican, in this case the late Senator Johnny Isakson, debunked the disinformation that Obamacare included "death panels." He knew, he explained, because he had coauthored a provision that was tucked into the Affordable Care Act that was being grotesquely misinterpreted.[76]

Isakson's measure allowed Medicare to reimburse doctors for time they spent talking to older patients about their *preferences* for end-of-life care. It did not, as anti-Obamacare activists and commentators falsely claimed, set up panels to decide who was going to get care and who was going to be nudged toward death.⁷⁷ As a conservative Republican speaking out against that distortion, Isakson did win some people over. (Although, more than a decade later, an astonishing 70 percent of Americans reported they were still "unsure" whether there were death panels.)⁷⁸

But credible communicators aren't always heeded; indeed sometimes they are pushed from their perch. When Liz Cheney, then a Wyoming GOP congresswoman, opposed Donald Trump over his stolen-election claims and the January 6 assault on the Capitol, she became a heroine to Democrats despite her deep conservatism on just about every other issue. But for Republicans, she was no Johnny Isakson. She lost her next election.

A similar approach is boosting "credible sources" of health and scientific knowledge, whether from our home at the Johns Hopkins Bloomberg School of Public Health or through medical and public health schools and systems across the globe and YouTube itself. This has begun, and it helps consumers encounter reliable information on major online platforms before they get the slime. For instance, when the RSV vaccines were approved in the summer of 2023, misinformation did bubble up, but it wasn't so prominent on mainstream internet sites. Someone doing a Google or YouTube search for "RSV vaccine" would first see several pages of information from established and reliable public health organizations and mainstream media.⁷⁹

Several academic and health organizations have developed projects, tools, and criteria to enable this elevation of credible sources, although it will keep evolving and being refined for some time—and may face an uncertain future in the changing political environment. The National Academy of Medicine has guided some of these efforts. In work starting in 2021, a NAM-convened panel focused primarily on US-based sources and nonprofits. A second stage took a global perspective and involved NAM, the Council of Medical Specialty Societies, and WHO. It established four criteria for source credibility: that the source had to be (1) science based, (2) objective, (3) transparent and accountable, and (4) equitable and inclusive. The idea is to help social media companies, researchers, and individuals have a starting point for credibility. But it doesn't establish that someone representing him- or herself as an expert online is actually an expert, or that all of their posts are accurate or even well intentioned.

As the expert panel itself noted, they "recognize that identification of credible sources may not be sufficient to ensure that consumers are accessing high-quality information, and social media companies may need to employ parallel strategies such as content assessment, management of misinformation, addressing health literacy, and culturally competent communication, and developing avenues for sources to self-regulate in order to truly address this complex issue."[80] That also means helping credible communicators learn how to be not just credible but understandable and accessible.

"If you've been labeled as credible, we are going to try to help you get better," said Helen Burstin, CEO of the Council of Medical Specialty Societies. Garth Graham, the global head of health care and public health partnerships at YouTube, concurs: "We [health experts] publish papers and accelerate careers but the public doesn't understand the information. We have been missing communities for a long time, and regardless of what you think of the platforms people use, that's where they are."[81]

Work is ongoing in the United States and abroad to extend this credibility designation to a variety of other health groups, including foundations, disease advocacy groups, and for-profit entities.[82] And the results can be seen on any screen—not just in that RSV vaccine search described earlier but in any health query on YouTube (and there are billions). The top "shelf" displayed is from credible, vetted authorities, like the layperson-friendly content from the American Academy of Pediatrics or *The New England Journal of Medicine*. It's not an anti-vaxxer, a conspiracy theorist, or someone's cranky uncle.

Nonprofit efforts can only go so far in boosting credibility—but given the political schisms in the United States, it's hard at this time to imagine a government-led alternative, or even a public-private partnership giving a cyber-info equivalent of a *Good Housekeeping* seal of approval. In fact, the first attempt to do something along those lines failed swiftly and spectacularly. A proposed Disinformation Governance Board that was to have been based at the Department of Homeland Security went down in flames in a matter of weeks after critics, including some prominent House Republicans, derided it as a threat to free speech, an Orwellian Ministry of Truth pushed by pro-Biden Democrats to censor tech companies and silence dissent.[83]

"Basically, everything you may have heard about the Disinformation Governance Board is wrong or is just a flat out lie," Nina Jankowicz, the designated leader of the short-lived project, later told NPR. "The board was quite simple and anodyne. What it wanted to do was to coordinate among the Department of Homeland Security's components—agencies like FEMA [the Federal Emergency Management Agency] or the Cyber and Infrastructure Security Agency or Customs and Border Patrol—and make sure that Americans had trustworthy information about issues connected to homeland security."[84] The disinformation board became a victim of disinformation.

Mobilizing in Real Life

Sources of credibility in the fight against misinformation are not limited to academic experts who can put out press releases. Many are rooted in communities across the country—faith leaders, business leaders, and local health care professionals. It's critical to mobilize such individuals in real life to counter misinformation online or in social media in the real world. This community-based outreach was considered to be key to fighting misunderstanding on COVID-19 vaccines among Black Americans, through programs such as the Black Coalition Against COVID. The coalition came together on Easter Sunday 2020 and was led by the National Medical Association, medical schools at historically Black universities, and Black doctors and nurses across the country.[85] It was also the key to the Made to Save coalition, which worked with 110 organizations to contact 5 million people and have more than 600,000 conversations about the COVID-19 vaccine in 21 languages.[86]

To Regulation and Beyond

There is growing recognition that grassroots efforts to share good information need help from policymakers in curbing the tidal wave of misinformation soaking communities across the country. Self-policing by social media platforms has been spotty; various attempts at content labeling, flagging, fact checking, and crowdsourcing have come and gone, and transparency has been poor. However, the US Congress and courts struggle with how, and how much, to regulate tech companies and still protect freedom of speech. Thorny issues include the definition of misinformation (and who gets to apply it), the level of transparency to be required, limits on algorithms, and the process of enforcement.

Help may come from overseas. The European Union's Digital Services Act, starting in August 2023, began holding tech companies accountable for what they publish. The law requires companies with at least 45 million monthly users to limit the spread of misinformation or face substantial monetary penalties or even the loss of the European market. Companies have to conduct regular risk assessments, subject to outside audits, and they have to offer individuals a way to turn off algorithms that offer content based on an individual's personal characteristics, including race and religion. But while the law's reach is broad, it doesn't affect all online communication, and questions remain about how it will work, in Europe and certainly beyond.

Even as global regulatory efforts have begun to move forward, some platforms have moved backward. Twitter's Community Notes feature is supposed to fact-check errors posted by users, but that didn't stop the proliferation of disinformation and hate speech under the management of Elon Musk.[87] No Community Note was appended to Musk's own tweet trashing the widely used Food and Drug Administration–approved antidepressant Wellbutrin. After a Community Note highlighted the errors in another Musk tweet, which had incorrectly linked the COVID-19 vaccine to the on-court cardiac arrest of college basketball star Bronny James (son of LeBron James), Twitter users voted to remove the correction, and it was taken down. As a result, millions of people viewing Musk's tweet would not learn that James's heart condition was congenital, and corrected surgically, and was not linked in any way to his vaccination.[88]

Today, a world of falsehoods remains just a click away, able to support any conspiracy theory and resilient enough to withstand most appeals to science and reason. Just ask Brandy Zadrozny.

Long before she was a network TV correspondent tracking a not-dead nurse, she and her husband moved to Vermont. She was in her 20s then, pregnant with her first child, and feeling vulnerable. She had never even owned a pet and now she was wondering how to be a good mom. She made new friends, including some who led her to fear hospitals—and vaccines.

As part of the podcast series on Dover, Zadrozny explained that after listening to her friends and neighbors, she made a plan to hold off on vaccination. "Planning my crunchy birth meant hanging out in online spaces where pregnancy and birth things were discussed. The second most popular topic was vaccines and my new tribe was just as critical of vaccines as they were of hospitals."[89]

Her midwife and pediatrician stepped up. They listened; she grew to trust them. "Patient and kind but adamant," she recalled. Her baby was vaccinated—and Zadrozny cried "because the misinformation had worked on me."[90] But facts had worked too. So had science. So had trust.

Now, with traditional media weakened and social media increasingly larded with falsehoods, a key question is where Americans can turn to find important information about their health.

We now turn to some answers, starting with a new breed of news outlets, nonprofit and issue oriented, that is emerging to fill the gap left by the loss of traditional media. These outlets feature solid reporting, in-depth analysis of policy solutions, and practical information people in different communities can use to protect their health.

• CHAPTER 4

The Innovators

After studying journalism and political science at Northwestern University, Alissa Zhu spent about five years working first for a small newspaper in Missouri and then for a somewhat larger one in Mississippi. She mostly covered city government and criminal justice, but her beats brought her into contact with many aspects of a community—and reminded her that being a reporter can be rewarding. It's an opportunity to learn something new every day, and a license to ask people questions. It can spotlight things that are wrong, and often hidden, in a community and sometimes even spark solutions. But even though journalism was Zhu's first professional love, she began to think about other career paths. It was impossible to ignore what was happening in the news industry across the country, at papers big and small. And the pandemic had begun, awakening an interest in public health. Zhu decided to leave her job and pursue a master's degree in public health. She arrived at Johns Hopkins University in the fall of 2021.[1]

It was fortuitous timing.

The Baltimore Sun had continued its slide and had just been bought by Alden Global Capital, a hedge fund. The *Sun*, as described in chapter 1, had been downsizing for years. The once stellar health team had been whittled away. With the Alden acquisition, more reporters quit. Among them was Andrea McDaniels, who had been a business reporter, an outstanding health reporter, and then a member of the editorial board. She had loved the *Sun*. But now it was time to go.

"I stuck it out through 20 years. I could have left. But you know, I really loved Baltimore, I really felt devoted to covering the city," McDaniels told our class. "As an African American reporter, I felt devoted to covering communities that weren't covered, to covering issues that weren't covered. But my last straw was when Alden, the hedge fund, became majority shareholder. And I just saw the writing on the wall. Looking at what they've done to papers across the country—they decimated them. Their main thing is the bottom line. Even during my last few years at the *Sun*, everything was about numbers." How many hits a story got online. How many stories a reporter turned out—whether the output justified the salary. "Everything about numbers, numbers, numbers. The bottom line."[2]

With her experience and reputation, McDaniels certainly could have gone to a newspaper elsewhere. But she and her husband didn't want to leave Baltimore.[3] So she too ended up at Johns Hopkins—not as a student like Zhu, but working on communication projects at the Bloomberg American Health Initiative, an innovative program that works across the country addressing overdose, violence, and other major public health challenges.

But the *Sun* saga would have another twist. A wealthy civic-minded Maryland businessman named Stewart Bainum Jr., who had come to understand and appreciate the role of journalism when he served in the state legislature, had tried to buy the venerable *Sun*, but when Alden outbid him, he had another idea.

He'd start his own paper.

"I served in the Maryland general assembly from 1979 to 1987. Back then there were six vibrant newspapers covering the sessions, including the *Capital Gazette*. Now there are two—the *Sun* and *The Washington Post*—and they have a couple of reporters each. As a legislator, I saw all sorts of shenanigans. Not all of them got reported—but a lot more then than now," Bainum told the Poynter Institute. He believed in that kind of scrutiny and transparency. Besides, he reflected, he probably still had "a public service itch to scratch."⁴

The nonprofit media sector had emerged a decade earlier and was now where some of the most hopeful and exciting trends in local news were developing. And that's what Bainum decided Baltimore needed. He pledged to raise or invest $50 million to back a new paper, giving it the time and space to find its voice—and its financial footing, envisioned as a mix of subscribers, advertisers, and philanthropy. Bainum called it *The Baltimore Banner*—a shout-out to Baltimore's role in the creation of the national anthem—and he opened it right in Baltimore's Inner Harbor. It is owned by the nonprofit Bainum founded to nurture local journalism in Maryland.

McDaniels was offered the position of managing editor. Excited at the chance to get back into a newsroom, particularly one that was going to grow after all those years of watching the *Sun* shrink, she accepted. "What's great about being here is that you can build it from the ground up. You can create culture from the ground up. You can create expectations from the ground up," she said. "You can build a staff from the ground up that looks at all the issues that are—that we think are—important now."⁵

And given that the *Banner* was born in the midst of COVID-19—and that Baltimore was a struggling majority-Black city with huge health disparities and poor outcomes despite having an abundance of hospitals—"health coverage will be an important part of that."⁶

Among the people the *Banner* hired was Zhu, who would juggle grad school and her new reporting job before going full time at the *Banner*. There, she would cover a number of topics—including food deserts, immigrants and immigration, and "creeping segregation" in a suburb nationally hailed for its harmonious race relations. Increasingly she focused on the opioid crisis. Her work caught the eye of *The New York Times*, which was starting an investigative journalism fellowship program for young local reporters. It was one of a number of innovative partnerships across the country aimed at bolstering local news. Joining that program gave Zhu time, resources, and mentors—at the *Ban-*

ner and the *Times*—to dive deeply into the major public health crisis of overdoses in her new hometown.[7] The work drew national attention, and Zhu and her *Banner* colleagues on the opioids project won a Pulitzer Prize for local reporting.

Nonprofit News

The number of independent news outlets is soaring, though not as fast as traditional papers are folding. Many of the new ventures are small, tiny even—far smaller than the *Banner*.

Not all will survive. But some have had outsize impact as they plug the holes left behind by vanishing traditional media—and introduce invigorating new approaches to the news.

When ProPublica and KFF Health News (originally known as Kaiser Health News) were formed in 2008 and 2009, respectively, nonprofit news was barely a blip. But by the end of 2023, the Institute for Nonprofit News had 425 members, with readers in every state of the country. Its 2023 report on "the state of nonprofit news" found that nearly one-third of the outlets were primarily investigative and just over one-third were primarily explanatory, with the rest covering news and events. Nearly half described themselves as covering local news; some focused on underserved rural areas. One in six had a single-issue focus, such as criminal justice, race, gun violence, food and agriculture, climate, or health.[8] Most are free—no paywalls. Several, and not just the big ones like ProPublica but smaller outlets like Inside Climate News and Mississippi Today, have won prestigious journalism awards, including Pulitzer Prizes.

This chapter will highlight some outlets that are contributing to greater public awareness of health care and public health. The next chapter will look specifically at nonprofits that are giving voice to communities—Black, Latino, Native American, women, and LGBTQ+—that have often been ignored. All are playing a critical role in covering health. ProPublica and KFF, both of which have grown into major media presences, have a strong health focus. KFF is exclusively a health outlet. ProPublica doesn't cover only health, but health, including global health, has been a cornerstone since the outset, partly because some of its initial hires were standout health journalists. Several are now editors, paving the way for the next generation of enterprising young health reporters.

ProPublica and KFF Health News

Charles Ornstein is one of these editors. He left the *Los Angeles Times* to join the fledgling ProPublica, at the time a somewhat risky and uncertain endeavor. He has no regrets. "Our sole mission is to do journalism with moral force," he told students in our class. "What that means is to expose abuses of power and betrayals of the public trust, and to create journalism that produces impact."[9]

Ornstein has done precisely that, at ProPublica and at the *Los Angeles Times*. He and colleague Tracy Weber, who would also move to ProPublica, worked together at the Los Angeles paper to uncover the devastatingly bad—often deadly—care for poor, mostly nonwhite patients, by then predominantly Hispanic, who relied on King/Drew Medical Center. Soon after their stories appeared, the hospital was shut down.

Ornstein, who later became a ProPublica managing editor overseeing local partnerships and initiatives, noted that the public sometimes thinks of investigative reporters as "decidedly critical and negative people," intent on slashing and burning. To him, ProPublica is the opposite.

> One of the things that motivates us from day to day is the idea—that we still believe—that if you point out something that isn't working well, that people of good faith will want to fix it and will want it to improve. That has been a model that has worked for us over the years and has produced sweeping changes across the country in individual locations. New laws. New policies. People exonerated. People fired. People jailed. Lots and lots of different things happen as a result of our reporting.[10]

Many of those "different things" involve health. "I've been able to see firsthand the power of health reporting and how people relate to health reporting because it's something that affects people's lives. So the response you hear from people to the reporting you do is overwhelming and it's what motivates me to do what I do."[11]

A former English major and math minor, Caroline Chen found the ProPublica health beat to be the perfect fit. She covered biotech for Bloomberg News—including, back in 2017, a look at what would become the mRNA vaccine technology. A native of Hong Kong, she was a child during the 2003 SARS outbreak, which was a backdrop for her to expand her beat to include a lot more public health, including coverage of the pandemic.

"I worked at Bloomberg for five years covering the biotech industry and had a fantastic time, including covering the emergence of Crispr and gene-editing therapies, the collapse of Theranos, and the West Africa Ebola epidemic. I was excited to join ProPublica so I could focus on investigative reporting and pursue stories in the public interest that weren't necessarily business focused," she said. "My role at ProPublica does not involve breaking news, so I have been able to devote more time and energy to individual stories. One example is my investigation of a heart transplant program at a New Jersey hospital whose focus on survival rates was warping how it cared for patients. That story required months of reporting, convincing insiders to talk to me and earning patients' trust."[12]

KFF president and CEO Drew Altman had long been a careful connoisseur of health news. By the early 2000s, he saw that it was failing. When there was a major health story, particularly with political implications, the big national media usually rallied to cover it. Local news, not so much. And when the story wasn't red hot, health coverage waned. Back then, nonprofit news wasn't a familiar concept, but Altman started thinking about what such a thing would look like, and why KFF, an influential health policy research nonprofit then still called the Kaiser Family Foundation, would be the right place to create it.[13]

With its public opinion polling on health and its multifaceted research on US and global health, KFF was already pushing out tons of health policy information and analysis to health policy professionals and related audiences. A nonprofit news arm could round that out, to inform not just the health policy aficionados but the American public.[14]

"I saw an increasing need for a nonprofit news service that could provide in-depth coverage of these really complicated health policy issues for the American people. Increasingly, the mainstream news industry was failing," Altman said. "I felt we would be able to do that, and that we could do that." It would both work institutionally and be a public good. "We would be not a policy research organization, not a polling organization, not a news organization, but a one-of-a-kind combination of all three. It was by having all three under one roof that we could play our role as an organization, as an independent source of facts and information on national health issues."[15]

The news program would be housed within the foundation and become an operating arm of KFF. But—and this was crucial—it would be editorially independent. Initially based in Washington, DC, and California, the journalists could report the stories that they, the journalists, knew needed to be told—not based on what Altman or other KFF leaders ordered up, and not based on commercial incentives about whatever clicks and traffic were driving business. KFF Health News didn't have to worry about that; it has been supported by a sizable endowment and, as it expanded outside Washington and California, by a number of regional philanthropies.

As the organization grew, reporters could spend days, weeks, or months on a project, not the quick turns that increasingly dominated strapped newsrooms at places like *The Baltimore Sun*. Memorable projects would include one in partnership with *The Guardian* that tracked every single death of a health worker during the pandemic, and a yearlong deep dive—with ongoing follow-up—about medical debt in America.[16] KFF Health News also partnered with *The New York Times* on a comprehensive series called "Dying Broke" about the cost of growing old.[17]

From the beginning, Kaiser Health News had a partnership model. It would have its own website, and it would include the news articles in assorted newsletters and summaries that KFF pushed out. But it would mostly publish them in partner "legacy" news outlets, both national and local—although as the nonprofit news sector developed, it would partner with them too. Other outlets could later republish them.

"We then had a distribution—not a destination—strategy as we started," said David Rousseau, who became the publisher in 2011 and has led the news services' considerable expansion. "We had a really robust and passionate inside-baseball crowd who followed every poll that [KFF] put out and every policy piece we did. But they were not America. . . . As we started the news service, to make sure we reached a mass audience with the reporting that we're able to do, we focused on placing every story with a partner first and then letting everyone pick up the stories for free."[18]

"That's another principle that we still have today; we don't charge for our stories. We're a public charity, and all of our stories are free for anyone to run," Rousseau added.[19]

Sometimes, in the early days, it took a while for stories to find a home. But over the years partnerships broadened, deepened, and became more agile. A story that published in a national outlet one day could be reprinted in Nebraska or Alabama the next, plugging in local news gaps. Early on, they also established a fruitful partnership with National Public Radio. KFF Health News reporters would team up with reporters for local NPR affiliates, and editors from both outlets would develop interesting local stories and narratives that would not otherwise have been told. They would be aired on both local and national NPR programs and be published online as well at KFF. In addition to producing terrific stories, the partnership also helped the local NPR reporters get a lot of training and experience in covering health.

The nonprofit health service started in the spring of 2009 with just a small group of experienced reporters and editors in Washington and California. By and large, it didn't try to replicate the coverage of the congressional debate over what would become the Affordable Care Act.

It did more to explain the broken system that the ACA would endeavor to fix and to explain what it meant for people, not just politicians.

KFF Health News expanded steadily, and a decade or so in, it began opening local bureaus around the country, not to cover the local hospital board, as Altman put it, but to broaden how they told stories about health in places like the Midwest, the Rocky Mountain region, and the South. "What happens in the agencies and in Congress is reasonably well covered," Altman said. "Our focus, and it is the bedrock focus of the organization overall, is what these complicated issues mean for people. We try to both localize and nationalize the stories that we do, at the same time. We take a complicated national issue that might be a Medicaid issue or Medicare issue, ACA issue or some health care financing issue and explain it in a local context so that it means something to people."[20]

They have also become something of a fairy godmother to other nonprofits and start-ups, not by financing them—KFF isn't a grant-making organization—but by listening, giving feedback, and making connections. Rousseau has served as chair of Media Impact Funders, which has brought together philanthropies interested in bolstering quality US media and the growing nonprofit sector, and he has also just had an open door to anyone with a good idea, or a pressing question, about how to get things done.

If ProPublica and KFF are now powerhouses, some of the nonprofits that have emerged range from small to tiny. Some focus on a state or region. Mountain Spotlight, for instance, was formed by journalists, among them Eric Eyre (see chapter 1), who left the once vibrant local for-profit *Charleston Gazette-Mail* in West Virginia.[21]

While some of the new outlets focus on a community or region, others have chosen a deep focus on one specific subject area, such as criminal justice or the environment or food. Most partner with larger media organizations, expanding their audience and inserting policy chops into legacy outlets that may be heavier on politics than policy. These partnerships, whether national or smaller scale, for profit or not, are broad. The Institute for Nonprofit News estimates that members' reporting was published or aired through 7,000 media outlets in 2022—including many for-profit partners—making their news available to millions. Much of it is free, provided as a public service, not as a vehicle for selling ads.

And many are deeply engaged in reporting on issues related to health.

The Marshall Project

Founded in 2014, The Marshall Project was the brainchild of Neil Barsky, who has been both a journalist and a hedge fund manager. He put in $1 million of his own fortune for each of the first two years and brought other major philanthropies aboard.[22] Or as Beth Schwartzapfel, one of the first reporters to join the start-up and one who would go on to do considerable health reporting, put it, "We were founded actually after a hedge fund manager read a book about this rogue sheriff during the Jim Crow era in Florida, and wondered how different the criminal justice system was now than it was then. And it was not that different. And [that] kind of seeded this organization with the idea that journalism could shine a light in places in the justice system where, if people only knew what was going on, they might be inspired to make change."[23]

The Marshall Project's mission, looking at criminal justice and the carceral system, was ahead of its time. Publishing on its own or in partnership with others, including *The New York Times* and *Frontline*, as well as with smaller, local outlets that want to broaden their coverage, The Marshall Project has uncovered harrowing stories of police misconduct, prison guard brutality, and systemic racism in the criminal justice system. Its story of how police failed to believe a woman who had been raped—thus allowing a serial criminal to keep on raping—won The Marshall Project its first Pulitzer Prize.

A few years in, the outlet started *News Inside*, a companion print publication led by Marshall Project staff who were formerly incarcerated, which is distributed in prisons and jails across the country. It began a video series, *Inside Story*, which is accessible to the large share of prisoners, about 60 percent, who are functionally illiterate (and to those who just prefer watching to reading). Already successful, the publication was well placed after the George Floyd murder catapulted police brutality and systemic racism in the criminal justice system onto the front page. The editorial staff has won praise for their ability to be passionate and insistent while still covering the topics with objectivity and rigor, as evidenced by the awards it has collected, including not only the Pulitzer Prize but also a National Magazine Award.

Health care—or, in prisons and jails, the lack thereof—has been a theme throughout. The outlet doesn't have one designated health reporter, but a number of its writers, including Schwartzapfel, have spent a lot of time on topics like the criminalization of addiction, prosecution of pregnant women who used drugs, the mental health toll of solitary confinement, sterilization, dementia, the impact of extreme heat behind bars, and of course the coronavirus pandemic.

Schwartzapfel draws inspiration from her first job out of college at a hepatitis and HIV clinic, which did outreach to the local prison. "This was in the early 2000s, long before the 'New Jim Crow' and long before 'mass incarceration' was a phrase that most people know—a phrase that your mom had heard of or that you could mention at a gathering and people would know what you're talking about," she said. Her work brought her inside the prison. "As a young person in my 20s I was so pleasantly surprised by how much I liked the people I met there and how much I thought, 'Man, if the world knew how much brilliance, sense of humor, and just how much humanity was trapped behind these walls, it would be remarkable.'"[24]

When she started feeling burned out by the public health work, she turned to writing and freelance work on criminal justice. Once she joined The Marshall Project, she reported on addiction, probation and parole, LGBTQ+ issues, and, during the pandemic, the impact of the virus on incarcerated people. "In the early days of COVID, everybody was locked down all of a sudden, and our editors were basically like, 'Go find out about how COVID is going to intersect with what you write about.'"

So she called the doctors she used to work with and people she knew in public health. They all said some variant of, "Hold on to your hat. Because from what we know about COVID, at this point, prisons are going to be incubators."

"People think that prisons are behind a wall and walled off from society," she explained. "But staff are going back and forth. And so if you are incubating COVID inside a prison or a jail, inevitably, those [staff] are the people who are going to carry it back and forth."

"The prisoners we were talking to were saying, 'Look, man, if we get it, it's because they bring it to us. It's not going to miraculously come from nowhere. . . . We are sitting ducks,'" she recalled. "It highlights all the public health problems that are inherent with prisons and amplifies it. That was really clear from the very beginning."

A collaboration between The Marshall Project and the Associated Press found that a half million people living and working in prisons got sick—and that was just in the first 15 months of the pandemic.[25] And the measures to prevent the spread of even more illness—lockdowns, quarantines that were in effect solitary confinement—added to the trauma.

The Trace

The Trace was founded in 2015 with support from the Michael Bloomberg–funded Everytown for Gun Safety and has since diversified its funding base. It calls itself the "only team of journalists exclusively dedicated to reporting on our country's gun violence crisis," including identifying solutions.[26]

J. Brian Charles, who had experience covering politics and policy in both for-profit and nonprofit journalism, was a Baltimore-based reporter for The Trace from late 2019 to March 2022. He described his work there as reporting on what "public safety means." At first, he recalled, he was "a mile wide and an inch deep." Then he and his editors decided he should focus on gun violence in one city. He would "cover the hell out of Baltimore." Charles wrote about criminal justice, and the police, and one failed effort after another to get weapons off the streets, only to find more and more deadly weapons replacing them. Increasingly, he began reframing how he thought about the ceaseless flow of weapons, beginning to think about the challenge in terms of public health.[27]

"I wanted to know how all those things affected people at ground level. And what I wanted to know most importantly was to get as close to the people who live in those communities and the people affected by this and the people trying to work on this issue," he said in 2022, soon after he departed The Trace to work on other projects.

He focused, in part, less on efforts to remove guns and arrest people—which wasn't making Baltimore safer—and more on the nature of conflict.

"There's a lot of criminologists, including ones at your place at Hopkins and other places in the country, who say that arresting isn't really working. Forget the constitutional part. It's not actually reducing much crime, and the data supports that as well," he said. "But what we have here more than anything else, we have a conflict issue."

His last story at The Trace was about a particularly distressing form of conflict—the murder of a community antiviolence worker "who was shot in the middle of actually trying to deal with the conflict between two parties." He was the third such worker in Baltimore killed in a year.[28]

Cops can "chase guns all day long." But Charles came to believe that unless the city grapples with the nature of conflict, it's not going to change much.

The Trace editors too had started thinking more about violence from a public health perspective. A few months after Charles moved on, they hired Fairriona Magee to become the publication's first reporter dedicated to the public health beat. Based in Atlanta, she created a newsletter about health disparities and environmental injustice titled *Tropes & Stereotypes*. As she plunged into her new beat, she spent a lot of time absorbing the research on public health and gun violence and interviewing experts who focus on that. She's been intrigued by the links between gun violence and other public health challenges, such as environmental decay and mental health. That "allows us to look at certain issues through a health disparity lens, to help identify how social, structural, and economic inequities impact certain communities. This in turn allows solutions to be more focused on the risk factors these individuals and their communities are being exposed to, and what can be done to address that exposure," she said.[29]

"I had to understand, How do we cover this topic? What's been wrong? And what needs to be done?" she said. "There's a lot of responsibility with this work."[30]

Food and Environment Reporting Network

Sam Fromartz, whose background ranges from being a Reuters business journalist to writing a book on baking bread, with some jazz articles in the mix, began writing a lot about food, agriculture, and the environment in the early 2000s. He also noticed that the freelance market was getting a lot more crowded as more and more talented journalists were laid off as their publications went through one belt-tightening after another. By around 2009, during the Great Recession, it had reached a crisis point.[31]

"There were just a lot of talented people who just couldn't get work, or were being laid off. So a bunch of us got together and said, 'Hey, what can we do about this?'" said Fromartz. Their answer was what would become the Food and Environment Reporting Network (FERN), which does both investigative and explanatory journalism about food, agriculture, the environment, their intersection, and the impact on health. Fromartz was a cofounder and for about a decade editor in chief, before moving back to a role where he could write more himself.

The first years were tough. They had a $10,000 planning grant, but the founding staff worked without pay initially (though Fromartz noted that FERN always paid its freelance writers and photographers competitive rates). It took off. FERN is still small—about a dozen employees—but it's had an outsize impact. Like most outlets these days, it has a website, newsletters, and podcasts. And it has partners; almost every major project is published with another, larger outlet, such as *National Geographic, The New Republic*, or, until its closure, the *Harvard Public Health Magazine*. "We knew with our budget, we couldn't drive a huge amount of traffic to our site. So we basically leverage other distribution channels to get the stories out there," Fromartz said.[32] That partnership approach has amplified the work of quite a few of the nonprofit newsrooms.

Much of what FERN does is directly or indirectly about public health. For instance, it covers the health issues associated with large-scale farms, which are "usually located in very poor rural communities, often communities of color, and there are a lot of issues with air pollution and noxious odors," he said. "There are health impacts in the surrounding community as well."[33]

FERN has brought attention to the harmful effect of soaring temperatures on farmworkers—and how so few states regulate things like access to shade and water. And during COVID-19, FERN's journalists were "kind of out in front," reporting extensively about the livestock workers and meatpackers who were becoming sick and dying of the virus in unsafe conditions.

"It was really difficult to get information out of the companies, who were initially sort of denying what was going on," Fromartz said. States weren't very forthcoming; the industry was pressuring them. FERN did a lot of reporting, including making Freedom of Information Act requests, along with a lot of "shoe leather reporting—talking to workers, which has its own challenges because most of these are immigrant and migrant communities." Language barriers were only part of it. "It ties into bigger issues we write about, which is the concentration in the food industry—basically monopoly power—that allows a handful of companies to sort of set the terms" for these workers.[34]

Climate change of course is another theme, including how it will affect the future of farming. (FERN's *Hot Farm* podcast looks at this from the farmers' perspective.) "It's not just the farms and how they produce. It's really the food we eat, and how will it be produced in the future. The intersection of climate and public health is an interesting one."[35]

Documenters and States Newsroom

Two of the glaring gaps in local news are coverage of local government, including long (and often boring) public meetings that have an underappreciated role in shaping municipal life, and coverage of state capitals. Governors and mayors may command attention from local political reporters, particularly in election years, but agencies and the legislature less so. Two noteworthy endeavors, one a form of citizen journalism and the other a robust and growing nationwide nonprofit news organization, are trying to plug those gaps in city and state reporting, respectively.

Documenters calls itself "people-powered news on your local government." A project of City Bureau, one of the early municipal-focused nonprofit newsrooms on the South Side of Chicago, it trains, and pays, both journalists and civic-minded citizens to attend public meetings of local boards, councils, and agencies. The Documenters, who are often the only media present, post real-time reports on social media and publish their findings via Documenters and other local news outlets. They cover everything from city planning and zoning boards to mental health advisory boards. As of early 2024, they had trained more than 2,200 documenters and covered more than 5,000 public meetings in about a dozen cities.[36]

States Newsroom was founded in 2019 to restore coverage of neglected state capitals—a local news trend described in chapter 1. "The level of government that has the most impact on our lives is covered the least," said founder and publisher Chris Fitzsimon, a former North Carolina journalist who also headed up a state-policy-focused publication for many years.[37] (States Newsroom took some flak early on for being funded initially by a left-leaning think tank; as the organization has grown, it has diversified funding and partners, but it still gets criticism from some right-leaning organizations.)[38]

The venture has grown fast. Starting with five affiliated digital news outlets in state capitals, it was on track to hit 40 by early 2024. It has also absorbed another state-focused online news organization, the Pew Charitable Trust's Stateline, which was founded in 1998, an early response as local coverage began crumbling.[39]

These affiliate outlets, places like the Alabama Reflector, WyoFile (Wyoming), and Source NM (New Mexico), typically have more reporters covering their state capitals—the governor, the legislature, and agencies—than the legacy papers in their states. And that's the mission: Cover state government, explain what it does, and hold officials accountable. That includes a fairly significant emphasis on health.

States Newsroom has a Washington, DC, bureau, which provides the affiliates with policy-rich national reporting on topics such as climate, infrastructure, education, and health, as well as journalists dedicated to covering reproductive health. "Every state has a reporter who covers health, mental health, public health in some capacity," Fitzsimon said. "Everybody touches on that issue."[40] Medicaid has been covered extensively, as have gun violence and the fallout of the Supreme Court decision gutting abortion rights.

Each state-based affiliate is independent, with its own editors and board, but they share and cross-post articles, without fees or paywalls. Their content can be reprinted, for free, in smaller and rural papers that had basically given up on delivering to their readers any content about their state government. The way the whole system is set up enables reporters and editors to spot trends worth exploring across state lines. One example founder Fitzsimon cited was a project on how several conservative states had quietly started making it harder, not easier, for ex-felons to vote.

"While we appreciate, support, and often do investigative journalism, we think the real missing link is day-to-day journalism," he said. "What happens every day is really important in people's lives and a humongous part of what we do—a giant part of our mission."[41]

Following the Money

ClearHealthCosts founder and CEO Jeanne Pinder had spent much of her career at *The New York Times* when she decided to take a buyout in 2009, without a clear sense of what she wanted to do next. That was around the time when the ACA was being fought out in Congress, and Pinder found herself thinking a lot about the "affordable" part of health care and about how difficult it was for people to make any sense of opaque and confounding medical bills. She took a class on entrepreneurship, won a $20,000 prize at a *Shark Tank*–like competition with a pitch to found a company, and was awarded a second $20,000 grant from the International Women's Media Foundation. "I figured like that was a sign from above that I had to go ahead and do it," she said. "So I did."[42]

ClearHealthCosts is an innovator in how it approaches health news, gathers information, uses data, and works with partners, both in the media and in the community. It isn't a nonprofit, although it does rely in part on philanthropic support and is available free to readers, without any subscription fees.

Up and running since 2011, the digital publication does just what its name says; it tries to make health costs clear. It began with finite projects, like finding out what mammograms and other procedures cost in specific cities and areas. It used a combination of crowdsourcing and more traditional reporting, along with a database that would evolve and support more sophisticated reporting projects over the years. Pinder described it as "something like a mash-up of Kayak and Waze," respectively the travel and traffic apps.[43] They initially focused their reporting on several dozen "shoppable" medical procedures, like mammograms, blood tests, and other nonemergency services that people can plan and comparison shop for.

They also publish guides and explainers for how consumers can do that shopping—how they can find out not just list prices but what it would cost them out of pocket, with their insurance or for cash, and other ways to navigate the system, like how to argue a bill or how to approach Medicare. (During the pandemic, they pivoted to working on access to testing, vaccines, health equity, and long COVID-19 but have since refocused on costs and access to care.) Much of it is done in partnership with other news organizations, both for profit and nonprofit, legacy and newer.

One of Pinder's favorite collaborations was a few years back with Fox 8 Live in New Orleans—a viewership quite distinct from the listeners of their New York Public Radio partners—NOLA.com, and the *Times-Picayune* newspaper. "We were at the top of the news—the 10 o'clock news, many nights," she recalled. The program invited viewers to take part in crowdsourcing price checks, then published pricing information as well as strategies people could use to dig out true prices and navigate the system. As its growth over the years has shown, it has been a big hit.

A decade or so in, hospitals by law now have to be more transparent about pricing. But they don't all comply. And the data aren't great. Transparency can be in the eye of the beholder. ClearHealthCosts has been incorporating available posted rates into its data when its staff think they are solid. That's not based on whimsey. They have a lot of experience slogging through and evaluating data by now. "We are journalists. We have a track record. We've won a ton of prizes," Pinder said.[44] And they don't just publish numbers. They use what they have learned about prices to tell stories—for instance, to give real-life examples of people who got overcharged and how they fought back.[45]

Cost isn't the only metric that matters; quality counts, but that's hard to suss out. Lacking other information, some people believe that the more expensive procedure is higher quality—even though this relationship is weak at best.[46] "We learned from a vasectomy pricing project, talking to men, that men really want the most expensive vasectomy," Pinder said. "They just really think that the most expensive vasectomy is what they have to have."[47]

Challenges Ahead

A hallmark of the new nonprofit media sector is collaborations and partnerships, sometimes among nonprofits, sometimes between the new nonprofit ventures and legacy publications. Several national organizations, including ProPublica and Report for America, are working with smaller regional publications, supporting young journalists for a year or two or while working on investigative projects. *The New York Times* is running the fellowship that enabled Alissa Zhu to do her opioids reporting for the *Times* and the *Banner*.

The growth, creativity, and energy in the nonprofit media world are impressive and invigorating. Yet challenges abound. At least at the outset, these nonprofit start-ups rely on philanthropies and foundations—some of which don't totally understand, at least not at first, that their money doesn't buy them control of the newsroom and what's written or aired. There can also be blurred lines and ethical challenges if a funder is supporting a media outlet concentrating on a certain topic—and the funder is advocating in that area.[48] This can be alleviated as funding becomes more diversified, transparent, and stable, and organizations like the Institute for Nonprofit News and Media Impact Funders help new outlets and new donors address the rules of the road.

Ethical challenges remain. There's a "need for more newsrooms to disclose donors and adopt clear conflict-of-interest policies to protect editorial independence and public trust," as a report from Media Impact Funders, the Lenfest Institute (which now owns and has financially stabilized *The Philadelphia Inquirer*), and NORC at the University of Chicago concluded.[49]

This is true for nonprofits as well as more traditional for-profit outlets, some of which are now fundraising for specific projects or programs--like the initiatives at *The Seattle Times* and *The Post and Courier* in Charleston, South Carolina, described in chapter 1. Several big national initiatives, including NewsMatch, through which major donors match dollars raised locally, have been supporting local news through philanthropy, and big organizations with a media focus like the Knight Foundation have also been helping outlets grow—or at least survive.

These nonprofits aren't "the solution" to the vanishing local newspaper, to the decline of American policy journalism, or to combating mis- and disinformation—or poor health outcomes in the United States. They tend to be in more urban and populated areas, so many of the vast news deserts remain vast news deserts. But these new outlets are not insignificant either. Not at all. As Zhu put it, papers like the *Banner* are "an interesting and cool" new business model, enabling her to see a future in journalism and to do work with meaning.[50] Moreover, in some places—including, as we'll see in the next chapter, in communities that have traditionally been ignored or underserved by the media—they are giving voice. And they are telling stories that matter. About government. About citizens. About health.

• CHAPTER 5

By and For

The Rise of Community Journalism

Dianna Hunt was one of the relatively few Native American journalists in big-city US newsrooms. She was—or so she thought—winding down a 40-year career in journalism, mostly in Texas. She'd been both a reporter and an editor at some top papers, including *The Dallas Morning News* and the *Houston Chronicle*. She'd been active in national investigative journalism organizations and had trained staff at smaller newsrooms on investigative projects and techniques. But in mid-2019, she decided to retire.

A year later *Indian Country Today*, now a multimedia platform known as ICT, reached out.

Indian Country Today was a 40-year-old newspaper that had gone through a series of owners, tribal and otherwise. The paper began to struggle financially, and various attempts to reinvent it, including a switch to a digital-only format, fell short. In 2017, the news organization was shut down and the assets handed off to a nonprofit. A group of journalists coalesced to try to revive it. Mark Trahant, a well-known Native American journalist and chronicler, took the lead as editor, bringing on a new president and other key staff. Hunt would join them.

"I got drawn in," recalled Hunt, a Cherokee Nation descendant and longtime member of the organization now known as the Indigenous Journalists Association. She stepped in first as an ICT freelance editor and then, in late 2021, with the pandemic raging, she became a senior editor. And after years of being, to the best of her knowledge, one of only a handful of Native reporters in the entire state of Texas, she was on ICT Zoom calls where "every single frame is somebody who looks like me." So do her readers. That representation is a cornerstone of trust.¹

Now owned and operated by the nonprofit IndiJ Public Media, ICT reaches deep into Native communities across the country—the 2.6 million or more tribal citizens and others who belong to tribes that haven't been officially recognized—and even more across the globe.

Hunt wasn't primarily a health journalist during her long career, but reporters can't—and she didn't—spend decades in the news trenches without covering health at least some of the time. Like when Hurricane Harvey dumped all that water in Houston, or when the first US Ebola case was identified in Dallas, triggering panic in parts of the country. COVID-19, of course, was a crisis of a different dimension, piled atop years of poor health, neglect, and underinvestment in Native communities. Reaching those communities, on whatever issue, in ways that were relevant, accessible, and on the right platform, was essential.

That, she said, is why she's at ICT.

Although aimed at a specific audience, ICT has a broad reach, she said. "What we're finding is that when serious, professional-level, high-quality journalism is done from a specific perspective, it's going to catch the attention of people outside those rooms."

Readers sometimes mail in a five-dollar check or a five-dollar bill.

"To hear 'I want to contribute. Thank you for being there. Thank you for telling our stories.' . . . I can't tell you how moving those things are," Hunt said. "Because really, these are stories that should have been done."²

ICT isn't the only media outlet serving a marginalized or neglected community that has been reinvented—or invented—in the last couple of years. New publications have arisen to serve Black, Latino, Native American, Asian American, women, and LGBTQ+ communities, among others. And as these opportunities have expanded, journalists and their audiences have followed.

The previous chapter described the boom in new independent nonprofit publications, many focused on public health. This chapter looks at a specific corner of this new media world, the growing number of news outlets that give voice to communities whose voices often go unheard.[3] Their ability to get start-up funding, often from foundations or philanthropies, grew in the midst of the Black Lives Matter movement, the George Floyd murder, and the racial inequities of the coronavirus pandemic. Those national events, or traumas, also helped them expand their reach.

These new media outlets weren't created specifically with the idea of countering the misinformation campaigns, often centered on public health or voting and elections, that malevolently target minority communities. But they have taken on that role.

Successfully fighting misinformation and bolstering public health requires restoring trust. And restoring trust requires representation so that readers, watchers, and listeners can read, watch, and hear people who look, speak, and sound like them. And that matters for health, whether the subject matter is practical advice on how to preserve Medicaid coverage or trying to fact check claims that vaccines contain microchips.[4]

Diversifying the Information Environment

For decades, US newsrooms were all white or mostly white. They covered communities of color sparingly and were often tone deaf, if not outright disparaging. In the early 1960s, that tone began to change, as reporters began chronicling the civil rights movement in a way that finally evoked and conveyed injustice—and TV, which was now in more and more American homes, was bringing the violent segregationist backlash into people's living rooms.[5]

The ongoing underrepresentation of Black Americans in mainstream media, however, was found to be a cause of racial unrest in US cities by the Kerner Commission, as the National Advisory Commission on Civil Disorders appointed by President Lyndon Johnson was commonly known. The commission concluded, "The media report and write from the standpoint of a white man's world" and have "failed to analyze and report adequately on racial problems in the United States, and, as a related matter, to meet the Negro's legitimate expectations in journalism."[6]

The doors of newsrooms and TV studios began cracking open to new voices, particularly Black voices. Eventually—it took decades—reporters and editors from underrepresented communities would ascend to the highest positions of American journalism, running newspapers including *The New York Times*. But for many journalists of color, some of whose voices are featured in this chapter, it still wouldn't be enough. In their view, the papers still covered the country, and the world, the way white people saw it.

Then, and now, journalists of color could take one of two paths—or go back and forth between the two paths one or more times during their career. They could work in mainstream newsrooms, trying to broaden the perspective and cover America and Americans more perceptively and inclusively. Or they could work for—or create from scratch—publications or outlets that served Black Americans, Latino Americans, Native Americans, or other populations.

Ethnic media has existed for generations—from pre–Civil War abolitionist papers to Tagalog weeklies to the thriving Yiddish papers of the early 20th century. But such media have historically struggled economically. Now, however, the rapid growth of new independent and nonprofit digital news outlets is revolutionizing coverage of these overlooked communities. In the new nonprofit sector overall, a little more than half the staff are white, and more than one-third are people of color (and some don't disclose race or ethnicity in newsroom surveys.) Some news outlets still don't have staff or coverage that is close to representative of the US population today, and gaps remain at the leadership level. But overall, the Institute for Nonprofit News said, "the nonprofit news workforce is more racially and ethnically diverse than many news industry peers."[7] And one major reason is that there are a large number of outlets serving specific communities.

The Black Press

Black publications have a storied history. *Freedom's Journal*, the first Black newspaper in America, was founded in 1827 to call out white racists and pull free Blacks into the abolitionist movement. "The only reason there is a Black press is 'to plead our own cause,'" it declared. "Too long have others spoken for us."[8] That pioneering voice would only survive for about two years, as the founders split and the one who retained control began pushing Black Americans to move to Africa rather than improve their lot in the United States.

The early Black press grew rapidly. By the start of the Civil War, there were more than 40 papers owned and operated by Black people.[9] Others would follow: *The Pittsburgh Courier*, *New York Amsterdam News*, *New Orleans Tribune*, and *Baltimore Afro-American*. Among the most historically significant Black papers, the *Memphis Free Speech*, where Ida B. Wells began her anti-lynching exposés, was shut down by a mob in 1892.

Some of these Black papers survive or have been revived today, though many folded or were ultimately swallowed up by white-dominated companies. The economic pressures that have damaged local news were felt even more acutely at Black publications, which have a harder time getting ad dollars than white outlets and have had trouble navigating the shift from print to digital.[10] Some that survived did so by turning to softer news, such as entertainment. By around 2020, one survey found 158 Black papers survived, mostly small weeklies, in 29 states.[11]

A half century after the civil rights movement, mainstream media had more Black and minority reporters and newsroom leaders; there were Black television anchors and top-tier Black editors. But the problems with coverage persisted. As recently as 2022, a City University of New York study found that in the first year of the pandemic, "nearly one in every four (23%) articles in Black media mentioned racism or related issues, as compared with less than one in ten articles (8%) in mainstream media." And in articles specifically about COVID-19 in that time period, Black media wrote "five times more than mainstream media on the disproportionate racial impact of the pandemic, and nearly twice as much as mainstream media on frontline and essential workers."[12]

There was far more coverage of health disparities, of essential workers, and of "maternal health, hypertension, diabetes, HIV/AIDS, and sickle cell disease." The Black media did a far better job of providing "historical context to present day challenges."[13] As racial inequity got more attention during the pandemic, some newsrooms reinvigorated the push for diversity, but as a *Digiday* report found in spring 2023, overall "media companies are still mostly hiring white people."[14]

So some high-profile Black journalists decided it was time to change. As Gillian White, a managing editor at *The Atlantic*, told *The Washington Post*, she had tired of being one of the few or only Black women in a newsroom "fighting for the lens through which you see the world to be seen." She said, "I wanted to, instead of sitting on a perch at a white institution and trying to occasionally get that work done, really do that work every single day." She would help launch Capital B—and the very first beat reporting position they would fill would be health.[15]

Capital B

Capital B was started by Lauren Williams and Akoto Ofori-Atta, former newsroom leaders of *Vox* and The Trace, respectively. The two women had met a decade earlier at another Black-oriented digital start-up. Williams and Ofori-Atta developed the idea for a nonprofit digital start-up by and for Black America. It would be based in Atlanta, with a national staff. But it would also build out local news hubs to cover major Black communities. Covering health for Black America was an explicit part of its mission, and they hired a national health reporter in time for launch on January 31, 2022.[16]

For Williams and Ofori-Atta, rebuilding trust among Black people who no longer cared about the news or had faith in traditional media institutions was foundational.[17] "Telling the right stories is an important part of Capital B and building trust with our audience is crucial to our Democracy and public health. Black people can't be left out of quality information or locked out of it by the paywalls of newspapers that don't cover their neighborhoods anyway," they explained in an essay introducing themselves and their publication.[18]

They continued, "News is important. What has been lost—and what's left—hasn't always been great for Black people. But having nothing is very bad for our future. What rises instead is low-quality or outright false information, sometimes that explicitly targets us. This has consequences for voting. And it has consequences for public health. When we started a news organization, we wanted to make sure we were building something that was going to fill the holes in local news for Black people."

The health beat was covered initially by Margo Snipe, a young reporter who had also covered health at the *Tampa Tribune*. At Capital B, she said, she would "dig into how racial bias in medicine impacts our lives and investigate inequities in the American health care system."[19]

She wrote about the pandemic, of course, but also about what the Supreme Court's *Dobbs v. Jackson Women's Health Organization* decision on abortion meant for Black communities, about maternal mortality, about menthol cigarettes, about mental health—and yes, about misinformation, including about birth control.[20]

The Native American Beat

When *Indian Country Today* was revitalized as ICT, public health coverage was not the main driver. In fact, the publication uses a fair amount of Associated Press health coverage. But when health has become a priority—including during the pandemic—ICT has gone all in, both in its reporting and in how it pushes information out to the community.

The need is great. Native Americans have far poorer health status than white Americans. Native Americans and Alaska Natives have faced, on average, life expectancies that are seven years shorter than those of US residents overall.[21] As a group, they are survivors of genocide, forced relocation, and cultural suppression.[22] They persistently experience higher rates of cancer, heart disease, diabetes, substance use disorders, post-traumatic stress disorder, and other chronic illnesses and infectious diseases than white Americans.[23]

And like other minority groups, they fell ill, were hospitalized, and died of COVID-19 at disproportionately high rates.[24] Yet Native American health gets scant attention in the mainstream press, and when it does get noted, the coverage lacks social or historical context. Illness is often framed in terms of "personal responsibility" or other individual solutions, disconnected from the social, economic, and historical context.[25] Nor is the Indian Health Service, which provides care to 2.6 million members of 574 federally recognized, sovereign tribes, well covered in the traditional media. That may be one reason that, despite the unmet health needs of the Native American population, most years the division gets less than half the funding per capita that other government health programs receive, including Medicare, Medicaid, the Department of Veterans Affairs—even federal prisons.[26]

Against that disheartening backdrop, one thing ICT did early on during the pandemic was create a 30-minute weekday TV show both broadcast and streamed. Like so many things in 2020–21, the show began in a staffer's living room, but it later expanded and became another way of getting life-saving information out about the virus to a population that badly needed it. That show was up and running before Hunt joined ICT but she recalled, "There was a feeling in the newsroom that we need to tell people more about how this is impacting Indian communities, Native communities, rather than just relying on the national perspective."[27] (In 2024, the program was shifting to a weekly format and was undergoing other updates.)

ICT met a major need. Mainstream news outlets employ few Native American reporters. Fewer than 0.05 percent—that decimal isn't a typo—of journalists at leading newspapers and online publications are Native American, according to 2017 data from the American Society of News Editors.[28] And they aren't covering "Native" beats or "Native health beats." There really isn't such a thing. As Jenni Monet, a citizen of Pueblo of Laguna, wrote in a 2019 essay in the *Columbia Journalism Review*, "Native Americans suffer from chronic misrepresentation and erasure by an established press." When those few Native journalists at mainstream news outlets do focus on Indigenous themes, Monet wrote, they are deemed agenda driven and "subtly de-legitimized."[29] And the news gaps are exacerbated by the fact that many publications that do cover Indigenous people are tribal publications, meaning it's hard to do hard-hitting accountability reporting.

One thing ICT prioritized during the pandemic was accurate, timely data—which was needed both to quantify the disproportionate impact that the virus was having on Native Americans and to catalyze action. Data gaps are a problem with public health in general, and it's often particularly challenging with minority communities. It was particularly acute during the pandemic. Unable to get reliable and complete data, ICT painstakingly started collecting its own.

"A lot of times on health stories, particularly in Indian Country, we don't have data—there is no data," Hunt said. "We knew that Native communities were being hit very hard by COVID. But there weren't any numbers that showed that."[30] ICT painstakingly built its own database, contacting as many tribes as it could. That's no small task given that there are 574 federally recognized tribes and about another 400 without official recognition.[31]

The Indian Health Service wasn't much help, at least from the publication's perspective. Sometimes people in the division reach out with information, but "a lot of times we are just bypassed," Hunt said.[32] In time ICT would build a pretty extensive database (and Johns Hopkins University would later incorporate some of those data in its widely followed trackers).

Those hard, bleak numbers might have had the biggest impact of any of ICT's coverage. "We finally figured out how hard those communities were being hit. By gathering the data and pulling it together and putting it out there in a credible way, people suddenly realized that hundreds of people were dying. And that they needed to pay more attention," Hunt said.[33]

ICT's days of near extinction seem to be over. The publication has a partnership with the Cronkite School of Journalism and Mass Communication at Arizona State University—where students have written some health stories that ICT posts—and as of 2024 it had bureaus in Alaska, Montana, and Washington, DC. It lets other publications pick up its stories, for free, as long as they give proper attribution. In late 2019, the Associated Press distributed an ICT story for the first time, vastly expanding its reach and bringing news of Native Americans to a far larger audience.[34]

ICT has also been part of a rural reporting collaborative under the umbrella of the Institute for Nonprofit News, which includes covering health equity among its priorities. One ambitious project steered by Hunt—who did not just do the editing but also the training and mentoring along the way—brought together about 10 publications, several of them either Native American or including Native Americans on their staff, to focus on economic opportunities including green energy. The collaboration has enabled them to collectively broaden their reach and resonance.[35] The Rural News Network, which now includes dozens of small independent newsrooms, not all Native, has made covering rural health care and rural health care equity a priority for the coming years, securing funding from the National Institute for Health Care Management and other organizations to build expertise.[36]

For Hunt, the ICT experience, through the pandemic and beyond, has been profoundly rewarding. "The ability to be able to reach people with the messages and the information that we have is something that I find very empowering," she said. "It pulled me out of retirement and made me decide this is actually fun again."[37]

The 19th*: Women, Health, and the Asterisk

Named for the constitutional amendment that gave women the vote, the 19th is a Texas-based, national news organization that covers women and gender. Its mission, in part, is to address the underrepresentation of women and LGBTQ+ people in political and policy journalism, as well as in newsroom leadership. That in turn influences "what stories are told, how the news is covered and whose voices are elevated."[38] The news outlet's full name has an asterisk after "the 19th," though, a reminder that not all women gained the right to vote then, and some remain disenfranchised today.

"It's an asterisk that we take really seriously," said Abby Johnston, an Austin-based editor, who had been a reproductive health reporter earlier in her career.[39]

Intentional or serendipitous, the 19th had a sublime sense of timing. Over the prior 20 years or so, a whole host of digital publications by and about women arose—completely different from the traditional glossies that focused on diet, beauty, food, and fashion. Most of the new outlets sank. The Supreme Court's *Dobbs* decision striking down abortion rights in 2022 and the domino effect wiping out or severely restricting abortion access in conservative states has invigorated surviving women-oriented publications, including *Jezebel* and *The Cut*.[40] But arguably nobody has covered the story of reproductive health freedom the way the 19th does.

At the 19th, covering gender, politics, and policy often means covering health—and vice versa. "Women, of course, are a huge audience for us. We write a lot about women, but we also write a lot about LGBTQ+ people," said Johnston. "People use 'women's health' as a shorthand for a ton."[41]

What the 19th has in common with other nonprofit news outlets focusing on a particular community or communities is, in Johnston's view, "that we're centering identity and central parts of identity. That is a very, very needed thing, especially when we're talking about health care reporting. It can be, literally, life or death." The 19th, she said, is able to "name that and take it into our reporting."[42]

Being based in Texas, the 19th, though only a year old at the time, was well placed to cover that state's groundbreaking law known as SB 8. The statute, enacted in 2021, banned most abortions at around the sixth week of pregnancy and included an extraordinary provision sometimes called "the bounty act" that let anybody—without being related to the fetus or the person carrying it in any way—sue anyone who provides, aids, or abets termination of a pregnancy for $10,000. That might include a cab driver who takes someone to a clinic, even if the driver doesn't know why the passenger is going there.

SB 8, said Johnston, was "a seismic story" for the new outlet. At the time, the six-week "heartbeat" ban, tied to detection of cardiac activity in the embryo, seemed too extreme to survive even the conservative Supreme Court. Yet what happened in Texas didn't stay in Texas. Within months, the Supreme Court overturned *Roe v. Wade*. Soon, half the states—including Texas—would have laws as strict as or stricter than Texas's six-week ban, albeit without the sweeping civil lawsuit provisions. And the country was embroiled in a deep, bitter debate over whether abortion is a sin, a crime—or health care.

"The ways to cover this are myriad," Johnston said in a conversation in the spring of 2022, after the Texas law was passed but shortly before the *Dobbs* decision came down. "We've mostly been focused on making sure that we're telling the stories of people who can't access abortion in the state anymore. What's happening to them, where are they going, what's happening when you can't travel anywhere?"[43] That included reporting in nearby Oklahoma, where residents of Texas were traveling to get abortions, until that avenue was blocked when Oklahoma too banned abortion with very limited exceptions.

The Supreme Court's ruling, and its ripple effects through the states, has been the dominant reproductive health story, but it is by no means the only topic the 19th's health and gender reporter Shefali Luthra has been tracking. "We cover gender inequities and racial inequities—and often those two are overlaid. They aren't covered at all at a lot of legacy outlets," said Luthra, who had covered national health policy for six years at Kaiser Health News (now KFF Health News) before making the switch.[44]

"We wrote about how the COVID vaccines being developed hadn't been tested on anyone who was pregnant. We wrote about the gender gaps in mental health conditions, such as depression and anxiety, and how the pandemic had exacerbated those disparities," she continued.[45]

(All of these issues became increasingly prominent as the pandemic wore on. For example, evidence would emerge—too late to help many people—that COVID-19 infection was particularly dangerous during pregnancy, and that the vaccines were safe during pregnancy.)

"Those are just frankly stories that nobody else had really written. And what was striking about that was we were able to find news that I think was really important. That continues to me to be important as a reader, as a reporter, as someone who exists as a woman in our society. And I also think that they served our audience. . . . This is news that matters to everyone," Luthra said.[46]

It's not that other publications don't cover COVID-19 or mental health or the debate about trans people (though not always from the perspective of trans people). But Luthra had the space and freedom to tell stories from angles that might not have been told, or might not have been told in depth or with such humanity.

"I was given a pretty broad mandate to say, 'If you find gender inequities that COVID has wrought, go ahead.' That is how I ended up writing about mental health disparities, about vaccines, about just what it was like to be a home care worker in the COVID pandemic or what it was like to be a teacher from a mental health standpoint."[47]

The 19th also tries to avoid what reporters call "parachuting" into a hot story and then moving on. That's when a reporter travels to a specific place, crams in a bunch of visits and conversations, with or without the help of a local "stringer" or "fixer," and then flies out again, often never to return. It doesn't make them a bad reporter, and it doesn't mean their stories are necessarily terrible. It's just how things are done in an era of limited time and resources.

The 19th aims to be a parachute-free zone.

"We are really committed to trying to stay with a story," said Luthra. Reporters get time to dig deep and follow up, even if that means a commitment of many months. For instance, before Luthra went to the border town of McAllen, Texas, which at the time had the only abortion clinic in the entire Rio Grande Valley, she spent weeks reading about access to abortion in the valley, and she talked to many people by phone. When she was ready, she went to McAllen and stayed several days. "I was not only trying to get a sense for what I had directly come to report—what it was like to access an abortion—but just to see what I didn't know, to get broader context about reproductive health care, about how different people in the community felt about abortion." And then she stayed connected to people after her visit.[48]

In other newsrooms, she said, she probably would have had to justify and explain why those stories mattered, or at least why they required such an investment of her time. At the 19th, "I never had to justify that, because it was so clearly part of our mission."[49]

The 19th also broadened its mission to cover the trans community, and health, specifically access to health care, became a big part of that. Again, Texas was at the forefront of the movement to restrict trans people's access to gender-affirming care. But the 19th has covered these developments as they've spread rapidly across the country and through the courts.

"The original mission of the 19th was to serve women in our society, and women historically have been marginalized, ignored, sort of treated differently because of their gender," Luthra said. "And if we are serious about examining that threat, we should apply it right to other people who are marginalized because of their gender. And there's been a really natural connection between anti-LGBTQ legislation, the particular legislative efforts to restrict access to health care for trans people, and . . . efforts to restrict access for people who might seek abortions."[50]

Latino News Media

Spanish-language media is nothing new; papers date back to at least the early 1800s, with *El Misisipí*, a New Orleans–based newspaper advocating independence for Spanish colonies, generally believed to be the first.[51] As recently as a few years ago, there were 558 Latino media outlets in the United States (excluding Puerto Rico and not counting local Spanish-language radio stations, which number in the hundreds). But many don't produce original news content.

The biggest sources of Spanish-language news are Univision and Telemundo—neither of which is owned by a Latino corporation. Many of the Spanish-language print publications are owned by larger Anglo media companies. Smaller ones tend to be independent and Latino owned. Most aren't well funded or well staffed, and they don't produce a whole lot of news, let alone in-depth coverage of health in their communities.[52] And in recent years, their audiences have declined, from the big TV giants to smaller weeklies, based on the limited data Pew was able to gather in its assessment of Hispanic media. Even circulation of *El Nuevo Herald*, the *Miami Herald*'s long-established Spanish-language sister publication, fell off, much the way English-language papers big and small have shrunk.[53]

More recently, there's been a burst of Spanish-language or Latino-oriented start-ups, most of them online nonprofits. Some are national, some regional, some local. Some are in Spanish; others are in English with Spanish versions available. Some don't fit neatly into any category: *Tostada Magazine*, a Detroit-based food publication founded in 2017 by a newly laid-off *Detroit News* reporter, focuses on the local Mexican community but has broadened to encompass many aspects of dining in multicultural Detroit (including how restaurants are addressing food waste and climate change).[54] It has partnered with other outlets, including through the Institute for Nonprofit News, to add a more national flavor.

"When I founded *Tostada Magazine* and started writing about Southwest Detroit and about Latino communities," founder Serena Maria Daniels said, "the response was immediate. People were starved for content that accurately reflected the community that wasn't a story about victimization or criminalization."[55] English is the magazine's primary language, but Daniels told us she's published stories in Spanish, Bengali, and Arabic, attempting to build a broader reader base for a niche publication.

But *The Nevada Independent en Español*, a Spanish-language publication within a publication that has arisen in Las Vegas—a metropolitan area with a big Latino community in a state with a rapidly growing Latino population—is intriguing and unusual.

For most of her career, Luz Gray reported in Spanish for Spanish-speaking people. Starting off in her native Mexico City, she moved to the United States in the early 2000s and spent the next 20 years working in print and radio, mostly for Univision Radio Las Vegas. Among other things, she produced and hosted a weekly community affairs show, *Contacto con Luz*, connecting Las Vegas community leaders with the growing and diversifying local Hispanic community.[56]

Gray still reports in Spanish for Spanish speakers, but with a twist. She's the Spanish-language editor of *The Nevada Independent en Español*, an innovative part of the nonprofit digital news site *The Nevada Independent* in Las Vegas, founded by the well-known Nevada political reporter Jon Ralston. The *Indy* is an English news site, but the Spanish site is not a separate publication, nor is it a translation of the English version. It's a hybrid.

The Spanish-language version has a definite Latino take on Nevada news—and does plenty of public service journalism in Spanish, including around health. But it's part of the *Indy*. Some of the best and most interesting Spanish-language stories get translated into English for that part of the *Indy* readership. And some of the top English stories get translated into Spanish, though of course many readers are bilingual and prefer to get their news from sources in both languages.

When the *Indy* reached out in 2017, Gray saw the potential and the importance. "That's why I was really happy to join—to get this information out in Spanish, information that is not always available to Spanish speakers." In a multicultural and diversifying region, "it's also about making the English speakers aware of those stories, these issues and concerns, that had been familiar only to the Spanish-speaking community."[57] And health coverage has been a priority, in English and Spanish, from the outset.

The approach—acknowledging and honoring differences but also bridging them—is unusual. Miami's *El Nuevo Herald*, for instance, has overlapping, but not identical, content aimed at the city's large and, generally, politically conservative Cuban American population. But the Miami papers in many ways mirror the separation and divisions in the community, not the growing interconnection.

Researchers at the City University of New York have found that other Spanish-language papers, particularly midsize ones rather than smaller community papers or weeklies, have English owners. Editors are often basically translators, adapting other Anglo-produced copy into Spanish but not deeply covering the Latino community. They don't produce a whole lot of news, let alone any in-depth coverage of health in their communities. And there are stereotypes aplenty, the same researchers found, with Latinos disproportionately depicted as undocumented immigrants—or worse.[58]

The Nevada *Indy*, Gray explained, is breaking down those stereotypes, building bridges—and also serving the unique needs of the Spanish-speaking people of Nevada. The *Indy* doesn't just translate stories, she said. It is "identifying the stories not only in the Latino community but in tribal communities, rural communities, in the whole state. So, we can talk to these communities and then bring up these topics and then translate them into both languages. So it is not really just the translation. It's identifying the stories and reaching out."[59]

These previously untold stories have a place in both the Spanish and English portions of the website. The Spanish-language initiative has also branched out to partner with a paper in Reno, radio stations, magazines, and online outlets "to extend the reach of our coverage and reach others who need the information." The *Indy* doesn't cover everything, but what it does cover, it does in depth. And its attention to its audience has built trust, Gray said, allowing it to become a counterbalance to the misinformation that has flooded Spanish-language media, before, after, and particularly during the coronavirus emergency.[60]

Gray said it's not just a matter of using the Spanish language or even choosing topics. It's the inclusion of voices. Voices from the community.

Voices from the public health community that arise from or have connections to the Latino community. "We are bridging gaps between policy and people, covering topics that the non-Hispanic audiences may have not heard before," she said. "We incorporate those voices into English-language stories, and we also feature their cultural and economic contributions. That's one of the main objectives. We have to fill that gap or create a bridge between these two communities."[61]

Because the news outlet has bilingual reporters, they can get to sources and experts in both languages, in both communities. Gray explained, "Sometimes we have, you know, voices or stories that are limited because of the language barrier. So with our bilingual reporters, we are able to get to those sources or interviews, and then we can not only translate the story, but also it helps to bring light to these stories." The Spanish voices incorporated in the reporting include both those of "ordinary" people whose perspectives and communities had been excluded and those of medical and public health experts whose inclusion can help build credibility and trust.[62]

The paper covers immigration, including the Temporary Protected Status for certain nationalities and the Deferred Action for Childhood Arrivals (a.k.a. Dreamers). It reports on culture, including writing about holidays, such as Día de los Muertos (Day of the Dead) and Fiestas Patrias (Hispanic Heritage Month). Education is also a major topic.

The Spanish-language reporters explain how the state legislature works—including on health care—to a community that hasn't traditionally had much of a voice there or much coverage shaped for them. "It's a totally new world for our Spanish-speaking community. They might be familiar with some names of public officials, but not really how the legislature works—or even aware of where the legislative building is in, that Carson City is the state capitol," Gray explained.[63]

Gray herself hadn't covered the legislature until she joined the *Indy*. "It's really helpful when we have journalists who are bilingual. Not only because of the language, but because we are able to start reporting on all these important policies that affect our communities."[64] That included a lot of the decisions Nevada was making at that time about implementing the Affordable Care Act, and the state's Medicaid program.

The bilingualism and multiculturalism were essential during the pandemic, both for informing the community and for building trust.

The Southern Nevada Health District and Washoe County Health District had daily media calls during the worst parts of the coronavirus pandemic, and the Spanish-language reporters were able to ask questions, push for more timely data, and reflect community concerns. It also launched a radio show and podcast, *Cafecito Nevada*, that devoted a lot of time to health. It let Spanish-language listeners hear firsthand from experts who speak their language. Among the guests was Fermin Leguen, a bilingual Cuban immigrant, who was the district health officer for the Southern Nevada Health District. He was also quoted in the news coverage. That created multiple layers of representation—the reporters and editors who looked like and spoke like people in readers' and listeners' communities as well as the experts who were from those communities and literally spoke the same language.

"I, as a journalist, can talk about issues in the show, but when the public hears directly from the sources, it really makes a big difference," Gray said.[65] That helped undermine or at least give a reliable counterpoint to the harmful misinformation about the pandemic in general and vaccines in particular that was inundating the community on social media. As noted in chapter 3, Latino communities have been targeted specifically by spreaders of public health disinformation.

As public health data became more available, the news outlet made them accessible to Spanish speakers too in multiple visual formats. Gray said, "People can actually see all these numbers and the information is right there. . . . It's not from social media. This is the data that we are pulling from the information that public health officials are providing to us."[66]

And it's all free. No paywall. "They don't have to pay anything to have access to the information."[67]

Creating Impact

Journalists seek impact. Some may want it in the form of fame and bylines and prizes. Others may want to know that they've changed at least their little part of the world.

There are many ways to create that impact. In a digital world, where news can travel far and fast, small papers can make a difference. So can representation.

That's been the experience of the reporters at the outlets discussed in this chapter. They are writing for their communities and providing a perspective that is often missed.

Luthra has seen the 19th's coverage shape how other outlets approach difficult or neglected topics. "The issues are really large, and if we can just serve those communities, it should be a tremendous victory," she said. "I genuinely do believe that these stories are just so interesting that they do break through. I mean the 19th is only a couple of years old, and our reporters are regular contributors now on national radio, on national TV. And I think what that shows is that things that we are writing that do serve specific communities really do have broad appeal."[68]

Gray has seen her work build bridges and create greater community on a daily basis.

Hunt isn't so concerned about the mainstream reader—ICT is not writing for them. But she too sees that when a story is "fully reported and put into context," it will find a wider audience, via the Associated Press or another route, and that "certain groups are going to read and understand and appreciate" it. But while that broader reach is rewarding, it's not the primary goal. "We write for the people we want to reach," Hunt said.[69] As a result, many thousands of people learn key facts and insights that can protect the health of their communities.

These innovative news outlets are working to keep their audiences from becoming information sick. The next chapter provides a playbook for health agencies, academic institutions, health care organizations, and policymakers to do the same.

• CHAPTER 6

The Playbook

Someone who fell asleep 30 years ago and woke up today would be flabbergasted by the changes in how Americans encounter information essential to their health. Odds are, as explained in chapter 1, if they went out looking for a copy of the local newspaper, they would be lucky to find one—and if they did, it probably wouldn't include its own health coverage. They might be surprised to find their local TV station part of a national affiliate, quite possibly sharing an overt ideological agenda with dozens or scores of other copycat channels across the country.

Surveying the national media, their confusion would not turn to relief. As described in chapter 2, other than a few national news sources that have remained intact, much of the national media has picked sides in the political divide. For every story they would find that really explored key policy issues, there would be many more on the horse race of politics.

Most shocking would be the volume of misinformation flooding everyone's phones and computers (and brains), across every channel of social media and communication, as detailed in chapter 3. At this point, our modern Rip Van Winkle might try to crawl back into bed, wondering whether the truth even matters anymore. And if so, how to find it.

Hopefully they would stumble onto new media, supported by philanthropy or subscriptions, that provide focused coverage for the general public or reporting for specific communities. These changes, discussed in chapters 4 and 5, would lead them to reflect on gaps in media coverage back in their own era, and even give them a glimmer of hope.

In the bygone days of the early 21st century, it was possible for high-priority health information to reach a broad public audience via press release and press conference alone. (Sometimes the press releases actually came in the US Mail.) Those days are gone. The playbook developed for the old information environment is out of date; relying on it is a recipe for failure.

This chapter takes on the challenge of what can take its place. The goal of health communication is to reach large swaths of the public with accurate information, growing confidence and building back trust. In this chapter, we set out the principles of a new playbook: for health agencies, for clinicians, and for academia. A separate, brief chapter follows in which we sum up some of what members of the public can do to protect themselves.

For Health Agencies: Rising to the Information Challenge

Before there were treatments or a vaccine for COVID-19, the only available therapeutic intervention was effective communication. Information made the difference between recognizing the threat of a novel respiratory virus and denying it; between wearing a mask to protect your loved ones and passing them the virus; between avoiding scams and falling victim to them; between receiving a life-saving therapy and rejecting it.

Many health officials became frustrated as their words of guidance and wisdom were ignored in favor of bogus YouTube videos or chat links—and as the health of their communities suffered as a result. As Renée DiResta wrote, "Experts generally try to create nuance. *Well, it may be true in some circumstances that.* . . . But in a world of 280-character tweets and thirty-second Reels, it's hard to do that and still be engaging."[1]

To rise to this challenge, our recommendation is for health agencies to focus on "the good, the bad, and the ugly"—promote the delivery of good information, minimize inaccurate and unfair news coverage, and counter the ugly misinformation and disinformation that threaten both life and health.

Promote Good Information

Not very long ago, a press release might have been all that was needed to explain the start of influenza season or call attention to a dip in childhood vaccine rates. Today, a press release puts the news "on the record" but doesn't meet audiences where they are. Health agencies need to map their media and social media environment and deliver key information across all channels.

An effective communications strategy should have at least five components.

First, provide context. Recognizing that few local news reporters are still assigned to cover health on a sustained daily basis, health agencies should supplement the news of the day with background information containing basic facts, cited to legitimate sources. Health agencies should also offer reporters a background briefing from someone who has expertise in the topic. For example, to supplement an announcement about where free influenza vaccines can be found, a health agency should explain what influenza is, why it can be dangerous, the evidence for the vaccines, and which health official or academic expert can answer questions about them. Particularly for larger national or regional public health organizations or institutions, virtual or hybrid news conferences are helpful because they give more reporters access to expertise. They also free the experts from having to respond to reporters' calls and emails individually. Johns Hopkins University, the Harvard T. H. Chan School of Public Health, and the Duke-Margolis Health Policy Center, as well as other leading schools and public health organizations, including the Biden White House, did this during the pandemic, expanding and democratizing access so a small-town reporter in Montana new to the health beat could have access to the same briefings as the specialized reporters at *The New York Times* and *The Washington Post*.

Second, coordinate with community leaders. Given the growing distrust in all institutions, including public health and health care, it is critical to share the work of providing important health information. Agencies should cultivate a network of people willing to talk to the media in the business community, in the faith community, and among other nontraditional partners. An announcement of a free flu vaccine might be timed with announcements from businesses that will host vaccination clinics, faith leaders who will encourage vaccination from the pulpit, and sports teams whose stars will be the first in line for shots.

Third, lean into social media. Americans are now spending several hours a day on their phones, getting information in micro-bursts from all sorts of sources, including each other. Health agencies need to be there too, rather than expecting audiences will also visit traditional, formal news sources to deliver the key content that constituents need to hear.

This means that health agencies should have accounts on all the key channels—which include Facebook, Instagram, TikTok, X (Twitter), LinkedIn, Bluesky, YouTube for the masses, and more for specific groups. Each account should have a voice, and it's possible to have multiple accounts with different voices, based on the audience. A simple example would be a Facebook account in English and one in Spanish in an area with a large Spanish-speaking community (or whatever language may be widely spoken in a city or region). A health department might also want to have a more serious Instagram account, which just puts out straight facts, as well as a more lighthearted and visual account that seeks to engage younger people.

Social media with video—such as YouTube and TikTok—are increasingly important and powerful. Finding the right way to marry message and medium may take some trial and error. Working with content creators in the community to translate formal news releases into approachable videos may be a promising route.

Fourth, consider new media. Innovative work on gun violence, if covered by The Trace, a nonprofit newsroom dedicated specifically to covering guns in America, could quickly reach a large and interested national audience. Health agencies should be familiar with The Trace and other issue-focused media, which offer an extraordinary opportunity for national exposure. Emerging journalism focused on specific communities offers a different type of exposure. A national agency worried about contamination of a traditional Hispanic food should reach out to a publication like the Spanish-language version of *The Nevada Independent* (see chapter 5) given its large reach in that community and focus on health.

Fifth, try to break into closed information groups. State and local health agencies should be aware of large WhatsApp and texting groups in their communities. Some may be limited to specific subpopulations, such as members of a church or synagogue in one part of town. Knowing individuals who are participating in these groups can help with disseminating information in key moments. For example, in Baltimore, these networks became quite relevant (and ultimately helpful) during measles outbreaks in the Orthodox Jewish community.

Correct the Bad

Because of dramatic changes in the news media, every health agency is likely to experience less accurate or comprehensive reporting than in years past. In most cases, errors will not be deliberate. Some grace is needed for the poor reporter who is covering the zoning board in the morning, calling school board members at midday, and fielding the health department's urgent announcement in the afternoon. It's a good practice to reach out to reporters proactively, offering to be a source who can explain health and science topics clearly.

Nonetheless, agencies should make it a regular practice to ask for corrections as soon as possible. An error is an opportunity to ask to meet with or at least talk to the reporter, establish a relationship, and be more available for the next set of stories. If it's not an outright mistake but a situation where the emphasis or context is a bit off, instead of asking for a correction, a friendly email with an offer of being available to provide context or answer questions next time is a good approach.

Not all errors are innocent. It may also be the case that reporters are pursuing stories to conform with their publication's agenda—ideological or otherwise. Among the potential responses are engaging intermediaries to speak to the publishers, developing and broadly disseminating explainer documents to be made available to people who are confused by the reporting, and holding briefings for community leaders about the nature of the coverage. In extreme situations, it may be necessary for health agencies to be proactive in calling attention to a pattern of errors in the coverage, using other communications tools at the agencies' disposal.

Another common challenge is how to overcome a journalist's devotion to a horse-race story. Rather than cover the progress of a new program or policy, reporters may focus on how embarrassing the failure of the effort might be to the elected leader. Instead of exploring whether a new initiative will save lives, it may be more titillating to speculate on whether the project will cost votes.

When an agency learns that the horse race is a reporter's focus, a starting point is to have a direct conversation with the journalist as soon as reasonably possible. The goal of the discussion is to explain how relevant it would be to explain to the public the actual health topic in question. A complementary tactic is to find other journalists to cover the content in greater depth, and to put out good information on alternative platforms.

Health agencies sometimes struggle to decide how much to engage with the media. Some advocate extreme care—either not calling a reporter back at all or drafting a statement and having it go through layers and layers of editing and fact checking and higher-up approvals before release. Avoiding reporters, however, does not stop a story from being written. It just stops the agency's position from being heard. Even a slow and careful response may backfire if the reporter is on deadline and has already moved on to another (perhaps less knowledgeable) source. Given the rapid pace of the news, this risk is far from theoretical. Statements need to be accurate, but they also need to be fast.

Is it possible to prevent bad news coverage? In some cases, the answer might actually be yes. Journalists are prone to pique when they feel like they are being stonewalled. Policies of information disclosure and transparency are not just good for open government. They can help build goodwill with journalists, which is always useful for a rainy day.

Counter the Ugly

It is now possible for a health agency to be releasing terrific content, working well with community leaders, and maintaining great relationships with local journalists—and still face a torrent of ridicule, attacks, and harassment. Misinformation and disinformation are so pervasive that no health communication effort, regardless of how innocuous, is safe from distortion. A health agency without a misinformation strategy is as exposed as a tortoise without a shell. This strategy should have at least the following four elements, some of which were introduced in our discussion of misinformation and disinformation in chapter 3.

First, monitoring. The agency should track social media and major chat groups for falsehoods, innuendo, and outright harassment. A regular report should surface key issues for various health initiatives and inform the development of communication initiatives across the agency. This report can piggyback on national monitoring activities, adding coverage of key activities within the agency itself.

Second, prebunking. Agencies should regularly communicate about the existence of misinformation and the murky sources of disinformation, in order to undermine messages before they even start to spread. If local academic institutions can contribute to debunking (or prebunking) efforts, all the better. Public health coalitions, both national and local, are emerging to spot disinformation before it takes root, so agencies should monitor this real-time reporting (or join the initiatives when that's an option).

Third, rapid response. When misinformation arises, the health department should consider responding proportionately. A single misleading or false post on X does not necessarily require a barrage of social media posts, media releases, and news conferences. It may only require a fact-check response on the same platform.

There is always a risk of spreading or amplifying misinformation while debunking it. This risk can be limited by describing the misinformation in general terms, not directly linking to its source, and directing people instead to a trusted third party for additional context. Instead of writing, "While many in our community are reading www.baldflu.com, much of the information there is not true. The flu vaccine does not make your hair fall out within 24 hours," a health department would fare better to say, "The flu vaccine is proven to save lives with the benefits outweighing the risks of rare side effects. Contrary to falsehoods now circulating in [town], the vaccine does not cause hair loss. Find out the facts about the vaccine from the university's site at . . ."

There is one clear exception to the idea of a proportionate response. Health agencies should demand responses to harassment and threats of violence. It is entirely appropriate for such direct attacks to be thoroughly investigated. In areas where attacks are common, agencies should work with legislators to increase oversight, stiffen penalties, and enhance enforcement.

Fourth, collaboration. When misinformation begins to spread on a grand scale, it becomes impossible for a single agency—no matter how well trusted—to contain. Speed is essential because as bad information spreads, it sticks. It's essential to engage elected officials, business leaders, the faith community, and others to provide clear, fact-based messaging and debunking to the public. The same networks developed to share good information can be utilized to counter the worst that social media has to offer. Indeed, in areas where this kind of collaboration occurred during the pandemic, vaccine rates improved.

The Communications Office of the Modern Health Agency

In the mid-2000s, the Baltimore City Health Department employed one person for media relations. She knew every key reporter for the city by name. Today, a successful communications effort requires a lot more, including the following:

- *Content creation.* Occasional press releases are insufficient. Modern communication offices should be providing regular content to key audiences on a broad range of important health issues across channels that span social media, email, mainstream media, websites, and more. Staff dedicated to this work are keeping the voice of the health agency strong even on slow news days.
- *Message development.* Offices should be engaged with national efforts to assess effective communication strategies for difficult issues, such as work by the de Beaumont Foundation, the Public Good Projects, and the CDC Foundation and its partners to support effective messaging.[2] There are also opportunities to join national campaigns such as the This Is Our Shot effort, which emerged during the pandemic.[3] As the strategies for rapid response against misinformation ripen, it will be even more important to stay connected with the work of these national initiatives.
- *Misinformation response.* A modern communications effort requires dedicated staff working to monitor and respond to misinformation and disinformation. These staff should be tracking national trends while monitoring local and state channels for emerging content. They should also be responsible for rapid, appropriate responses and briefing of senior officials during crises. National resources exist to support this effort,

such as the KFF *Health Misinformation Monitor*, and as we write this, more real-time monitoring and rapid-response initiatives are being developed.[4]

- *Network development.* The communications office should be constantly building relationships across government agencies, businesses, the faith community, and other key constituencies in civil society. For large agencies, at least one person should be devoted full time to finding, listening to, and supporting a network of communication partners and external validators, who can help share messages with audiences.

For Academic Institutions: Sharing Insights Based in Evidence

Academic institutions have direct access to research and evidence. They have firsthand training to analyze, to question, to debunk, to bolster, and to advise. In many communities, they may be more trusted than politicians, the media, and big business.[5] They also bring a huge range of disciplines together in one institution.

These advantages create a responsibility for academic institutions to share their knowledge and expertise to promote health. But they too must be mindful of the perilous environment and strategic about how and where they share their knowledge.

Academic institutions should develop content and distribution channels to communicate directly to audiences, including the media, public health agencies, clinicians, policymakers, and the public. And the content on these channels needs to meet the needs of those audiences, in substance and in style.

This isn't easy. It requires investing in communications within the institution. It requires encouraging and training faculty to be a part of that operation. It requires supporting the institution's faculty and leadership with talented and trained communications staff, including strategists, writers, editors, and designers. On top of that, the team needs expertise in media relations, community relations, stakeholder relations, audience development, and crisis management.

After the institution has made external communication a priority, and set it up and staffed it appropriately, the focus becomes the day-to-day work of getting each communication right.

The topics in the world of health are both wide ranging and fine pointed. What an academic institution has knowledge about is vast—both new and known, timely and timeless.

It can be hard to know where to focus. Generally, academic institutions can decide where to focus their communications resources and energy by considering the following:

- what topics are urgent right now where health information can make a difference (e.g., getting vaccinated during respiratory virus season)
- what topics the institution has new or unique knowledge about (e.g., a recent report that finds, somewhat surprisingly, that narrowing travel lanes on roads could save lives)[6]
- where the organization's evidence and expertise could be particularly helpful in addressing misinformation or, if not outright misinformation, in bringing facts and clarity to topics that lack clear and definitive information (e.g., how to understand the risks of myocarditis with the COVID-19 vaccine).

Once a topic is chosen, there are several key steps to get the words and presentation right.

First, determine the key messages. Ground them in evidence. Articulate the messages in language audiences can easily understand. Simplify the language as much as possible, as jargon obscures meaning and creates skepticism.

Second, include actionable calls to action. Communicate insights and recommendations that audiences can act on. For policymakers, it could be policy change. For the public, it could be an individual action they can take.

Third, be transparent. Acknowledge limitations, gaps in evidence, and potential critiques. By recognizing, rather than ignoring, opposing views or contrasting evidence, researchers earn trust and gain credibility. They acknowledge important complexities and nuances. But they need to do so without obscuring the key messages and calls to action.

Fourth, vary formats and platforms. Deploy a diverse toolbox of tactics in strategic ways that match the content and the audience's needs. For example, for emerging topics and science, a media briefing or a podcast episode allows a more thorough discussion than a brief web article. For quick-turn news developments, a social post or podcast episode may come together more quickly than a comprehensive report. Do not expect one format or platform to work for all.

Fifth, embrace repetition, repurposing, and resurfacing. Repeat and reframe many messages in different ways. Covering each topic once is simply not enough. Repurpose content from one source to another—for example, turning a podcast transcript into a Q&A article, or an event audio into a podcast. Resurface content multiple times, whether because it is relevant to new developments or simply because it merits another turn in the spotlight.

Let's look at this approach in practice, using the example of our home institution.

The Johns Hopkins Bloomberg School of Public Health seeks to be a go-to trusted source of public health information for a broad audience. It seeks to make its public health research, evidence, and solutions accessible to and discoverable by anyone. That means putting the content online, in ways that turn up in social feeds and search results, and in packages that lay audiences can understand.

One of the Bloomberg School's most successful campaigns during the COVID-19 pandemic guided friends and family—the ultimate trusted local messengers—about how to talk to their loved ones about getting vaccinated. The idea was that the academic institution would empower its audiences to talk to *their* networks, and that that would be more persuasive and effective for many ultimate audiences than hearing directly from the academic institution.

The campaign, "How to Talk to Friends and Family About COVID-19 Vaccines," lived on social media, in English and Spanish, with a supporting article on the Bloomberg School's website.[7] Bloomberg School faculty provided the substance—scientific evidence and research-grounded interpersonal talking points addressing vaccine hesitancy. The Bloomberg School's communications and marketing team provided the style—writing, design, skillful edits, and translation.

On its first run organically, the campaign reached more than 750,000 users across three social platforms. Additionally, multiple local health departments—from New Jersey, to California, to Alaska—asked for permission to share content with their local audiences.

The Bloomberg School also collaborated with Meta (Facebook) to run ad campaigns promoting the content. It used Meta's Brand Lift Survey tool to test how effective the campaign was in improving vaccine confidence and knowledge. Two studies, one in English and one in Spanish, demonstrated statistically significant positive survey responses when users were asked about the importance of vaccines, knowledge of vaccination efficacy, and ad recall, compared with users who did not receive the content. The campaign helped reach millions of people, thousands of whom took actions such as sharing the content with others to protect their health. The media wasn't involved here and didn't need to be.

The highly charged issue of gun violence prevention offers another example. The Center for Gun Violence Solutions at Johns Hopkins conducts research to identify solutions proven to reduce the risk of gun violence. Among them is this relatively straightforward recommendation: "Safely storing firearms can reduce gun injuries and deaths, and is supported by researchers, health care professionals, and gun owners alike."[8] Survey research conducted by the center also found that more than half of US gun owners do not safely store their guns.[9]

The Bloomberg School's communications team sought to promote this straightforward recommendation. The team put together a scannable Q&A explainer on the topic and another article to encourage people to talk openly about the importance of safe gun storage.[10] They added a highly visual social campaign focused on encouraging parents to ask other parents about guns in the home when setting up a playdate.[11]

The school paid to boost the content on social media so it would show up for certain target audiences. They also translated the content into Spanish.

Over a six-week span, the content saw more than 3 million impressions.

These examples show how content from academic institutions can travel outside the ivory tower and have an impact on the "real world." They can also provide helpful models for the communications by public health groups, clinicians, and other messengers discussed in this chapter to emulate or amplify.

For Clinicians and Health Care Organizations: Training Thyself

Clinicians generally fall into two camps. There are those who are already aware that their patients are exposed to torrents of falsehoods about their health and safety, in an information environment weakened by the loss of traditional media. And then there are those who will soon learn.

The initial instinct of many clinicians is to rely on their authority and training and simply tell patients the truth. Call this the "There are no microchips in the COVID-19 vaccine" strategy, and the good news is, it can work. Patients who trust their physicians and other health care providers may actually listen to their advice, notwithstanding the misinformation and disinformation coming their way on Facebook, TikTok, WhatsApp, and other platforms.

But not always. One of the enduring frustrations of the COVID-19 pandemic were stories of clinicians stunned that their patients believed outlandish lies over the information provided by health professionals standing right in front of them. "If you've got a gunshot wound or stab wound or you're having a heart attack, you want to see me in the emergency department," one physician told the Associated Press. "But as soon as we start talking about a vaccine, all of a sudden I've lost all credibility."[12] The erosion of trust in the health care system and in health care providers is far deeper than many health professionals realize. And millions of Americans don't have a close and ongoing relationship with a health provider, so that trust doesn't develop in the first place.

Many health professionals take the fight against misinformation to social media. As one nurse said in a recent study from the University of Texas, "Because people look to us as experts and if we are not standing up and making clear what is accurate information and what's not, I personally feel that we're not doing our job."[13]

But when clinicians engage on social media, the experience can be immensely frustrating. Debate over medical facts can undermine confidence that there is any right answer and move patients further away from protecting themselves. In October 2020, Canadian and North Carolina researchers conducted an experiment using 500 US residents. They were divided into four groups: one exposed to misinformation about masking, one also exposed to a debunking of that misinformation, and two exposed to more extended back-and-forth about the misinformation. While the debunking alone was helpful, the researchers found "extended exposure to false claims and debunking attempts appear to weaken the belief that there is an objectively correct answer . . . which leads to less positive reactions towards masking as the prescribed behavior."[14]

Making matters worse, US physicians and nurses have reported harassment and bullying on social media when they try to stand up for science. One physician told the Texas researchers, "Every single time you post about vaccines you will get harassed if your platform is large enough that people will see it. . . . I've had people come on to my Instagram and comment on pictures of my children saying they look vaccine-injured and that I am a child abuser and that I'm in bed with big pharma and my kids should be taken away."[15]

The result is that clinicians may be tempted to tune out or give up. If patients are going to fall prey to misinformation, the thinking goes, that's on them. But every time a patient turns away from a necessary vaccine or treatment, there is something lost—not only for public health but also for the special role of the clinician-patient relationship in society.

There's a better approach—and it starts with the basics. Before jumping to rebutting the latest conspiracy theory, clinicians can model a good information diet. If there is a good local source of news, consider subscribing and leaving print versions out for patients. Print out articles from specialty news sites, such as Capital B or ICT, and provide them to patients who might be interested. Have handy key information sheets from trusted local and state health departments and the Centers for Disease Control and Prevention. It may help to personalize the source of public health information for patients: the local health agency is not a nameless, faceless bureaucracy; it's led by someone we can trust who has lived in the community for 25 years.

A second step is to seek out training at professional meetings, where clinicians can learn about behavioral theories that inform more effective communication with patients. In a research paper, Johns Hopkins professor Daniel Salmon and his colleagues summarized some of these theories. These included:

- tailoring theory, which suggests it's important to "get the right message to the right person from the right messenger" and acknowledges that people who are skeptical require a different message from those who are already confident in the recommended course of action;
- narrative theory, which recommends that clinicians use personal stories about how an illness such as COVID-19 affected them;
- timing inoculation theory, which calls for providing "a small dose of arguments 'from the other side' the audience is likely to encounter, so they are more able to resist the message when subsequently exposed";
- health belief model, which uses animation and metaphors to make the benefits of the recommended action clear; and

- psychological reactance theory, which frames animation and messages "as information to help people make their own decisions (rather than pressure to get a vaccine)."[16]

In one study, Salmon and colleagues gave pregnant patients a survey about their attitudes on recommended vaccines. Those "who already intended to vaccinate received a short message reinforcing the value of vaccination." But those with concerns received messages connecting to shared values without reinforcing myths. The researchers told women worried about vaccine ingredients that "it's understandable that she would want to be careful with everything that goes in her body when pregnant" rather than "it's understandable that she would be concerned about vaccine ingredients." The result was a two-thirds reduction in requests for additional information and a 61 percent increase in vaccination.[17]

Like any clinical skill, talking to patients requires training and practice. During the COVID-19 pandemic, one of the authors volunteered extensively with a local public health department on the vaccination team. Part of his job was asking people in the community whether they wanted to be vaccinated. He found that the right question to ask a vaccine-skeptical person was not, "Why don't you want to be vaccinated?" but rather, "If you do get vaccinated, who would you get vaccinated for?" The latter question often opened up conversation about concern for chronically ill parents, children, and friends—and led to a decision to be vaccinated.

A third step for clinicians engaging with misinformation is to join forces, rather than go at it alone. In Chicago, during the pandemic, the Illinois Medical Professionals Action Collaborative Team came together across multiple institutions to develop "myth debunking" materials and a "vaccine information series" of infographics, write more than 50 op-eds, and support more than 200 news stories. The effort included creating, in English and Spanish, "train the trainer" videos to teach Chicago librarians how to communicate reliably about vaccines. The organizers found that "although individual efforts remain important . . . this novel method of collective advocacy with a community or place-based approach has the ability to amplify and leverage evidence-based information on social media and other platforms, with the possibility of timely change for the public in real time."[18]

It's critical that clinicians receive support from their organizations to do this work. Health systems, hospitals, large physician practices, and others should support training and collaboration opportunities in addressing patient concerns that are based on misinformation. Organizations should provide branded information on key topics, demonstrating, for example, that the local hospital does support recommended vaccinations. And when controversy comes, as it will, these organizations should stand up for their clinicians and for the truth, rather than try to duck exposure, as happened with the case of Tiffany Dover, the "dead" nurse in chapter 3, whose hospital refused to comment about how she was doing and, according to her family members, even told her to stay quiet, providing rocket fuel for mistruths to circulate.

For Policymakers: Taking Action

A tectonic shift in the information environment has taken place without a major policy response. Some of the trends described in this book were set in motion by policy that permitted the concentration of media, allowing large companies to purchase hundreds of television stations, radio outlets, and newspapers. Yet members of Congress at times appeared more eager to curry favor with media and technology companies than to reckon with ongoing harm to communities.

Policymakers have many opportunities to do better. The Federal Communications Commission can step in and try to reverse or at least slow down the concentration of media. Lawmakers can also act on assorted proposals, some dating back a decade, to create tax breaks that give local newspapers some breathing room. A few states have come up with programs to bolster local media, without trampling on its independence. Others should follow.[19] And there have been moves, in the United States and overseas, to require tech companies to pay news outlets for content.

Congress can take action on social media, setting guard rails on algorithms, or at the least facilitating efforts in civil society to address them. Recently, Senator Elizabeth Warren and Senator Lindsey Graham proposed the idea of an independent, bipartisan regulator for technology and social media companies "to prevent online harm, promote free speech and competition, guard Americans' privacy and protect national security."[20] Such a regulator could, in theory, track data about the impact of technology (including artificial intelligence), develop expertise about the harms of social media, and fashion a regulatory approach that balances the benefits and harms for society. With respect to artificial intelligence, an empowered regulator could make sure that news organizations are fairly compensated for their content, while limiting the ability to mimic legitimate news sources. In our view, given the immense and growing threats within our information environment, this is the kind of substantive response the nation needs.

Ultimately, we need a movement of "information environmentalists"—health officials, clinicians, academic experts, policymakers, and citizens—to clean up the mess that is obscuring the truth and undermining health. This requires simultaneously countering the forces creating harm while providing the moral equivalent of clean air and water—good information that helps people to protect themselves, their families, and their communities.

• CHAPTER 7

Protecting Yourself—and Others

The internet is an amazing resource, a fountain of infinite knowledge and fascination. It's also a cesspool of lies that can confuse us, mislead us, or harm us. You likely know people in your friend circle, family, or workplace who are at risk for becoming information sick—or are already there.

This brief chapter gives you some tips and tools to help them and protect yourself. The goal is to enjoy the benefits of technology without inadvertently spreading and amplifying anything incorrect or downright malicious. The chapter includes some fact-checking and debunking tools, as well as some inoculation or prebunking tools that aim to fortify our defenses against disinformation. We also include resources for improving media literacy, and a few tips on how to respond to things you see online with your common sense, not your emotional hot spots.

First, Read the News

Most of us are busy, distracted, pulled in a dozen directions. We get snippets of news all day—and often all night—mostly through social media or news sites on our phones, which we glance at quickly. But many of us no longer set aside time to really read (or listen, or watch) the news. The best way to protect yourself from misinformation is to pay attention to information. There are still many free or inexpensive news sources, including consumer websites of major national/international wire services like Reuters and the Associated Press. Many of the innovators we've highlighted in this book are free, and digital-only subscriptions are often affordable. Some outlets let you share a purchased subscription with someone else (and it doesn't have to be a family member). Subscriptions may be discounted for students and teachers. And many of the big national media companies that do charge for subscriptions still offer newsletters and podcasts for free.

We also think it's important to get outside your media bubble. At least now and then, take a look at something that isn't part of your normal media diet or worldview. Our country is deeply, harmfully, painfully divided. Seeing what the other half is hearing—even if it raises your blood pressure or reminds you of a particularly awful extended family Thanksgiving—is also part of being well informed.

Check Out Fact Checking

Even the best media routine won't save you from the misinformation and disinformation surging throughout society. That's why it helps to be familiar with fact-checking resources. Some focus more on politics, but they do address health and science, partly because health and science are now so woven into our politics.

Two of the best are PolitiFact, run by the Poynter Institute, a nonprofit journalism research and educational organization, and FactCheck.org, run by the Annenberg Public Policy Center of the University of Pennsylvania.[1] The latter has a section called SciCheck, which focuses on health, medicine, and science, and it also has a "Viral Spiral" feature that helps people detect misinformation and made-up stories. Both can be found on the home page.

Factchequeado, launched by organizations in Spain and Argentina, counters misinformation in the US Hispanic and Latino communities.[2] (The website is in English and Spanish.) There are also a number of fact-checking organizations overseas. More than 100 organizations work with the International Fact-Checking Network, also at Poynter.[3]

Major news outlets like the Associated Press and *The Washington Post* run their own fact-checking features, and much of that is viewable without a paid subscription.[4]

Of course, the people who are most likely to wholeheartedly embrace disinformation are not the ones most likely to check out these sites, or to be easily persuaded by them. But for the rest of us, when trying to sort out truth from slickly packaged and pervasive untruth, the tools can be quite helpful. Remember that disinformation often contains a smidgen of truth, or it may use a legitimate research study as a starting point and then distort it. Those factual tidbits are lures, pulling us into what we think is genuine. It's a bit like having real chocolate chips enticing us to eat a poisonous cookie. The fact-checking sites can prevent that first bite—or at least the second.

Inoculate Yourself

Inoculation, often in the form of an online game, helps us understand and build resistance to the ways that people and organizations (or hostile countries) behind the online misinformation are trying to manipulate us—and helps us to not fall victim to that.[5] For many of these games, the way to win is to go viral—and that requires messaging that you may think is so far out there that no one will fall for it. That's the point; people do fall for it, and these games teach you how not to be among them, "inoculating" you so you can better resist "infection" by disinformation.

Often developed by universities that are researching disinformation and how to combat it, the games illustrate how fear, resentment, outrage, aggrievement, and similar negative emotions propel and reinforce the spread of disinformation. There are quite a few such games out there, among them *Bad News*, *Harmony Square*, *Go Viral!*, *Spot the Troll*, and *Cranky Uncle* (which focuses on climate). These games are frequently updated. You can search online for the latest iterations and new entries. They only take a few minutes to play, and they also work well as group activities in a classroom or similar setting.

Build Your News Literacy

A number of programs have been developed to improve news literacy, a form of critical thinking that is crucial for both public health and larger democratic institutions. Some are designed to be used in classrooms, a form of civics for the 21st century. Others can be used in group settings or for individuals. The News Literacy Project, for instance, has tracks for educators and for everyone else.[6] MediaWise, another Poynter project, is good for any age but has particular salience for teens, and there's a version for older people who are particularly vulnerable to misinformation and scams.[7] Trusting News isn't about helping consumers of media to improve their literacy; it is an organization dedicated to helping news outlets rebuild trust with their readers, listeners, and viewers. It's designed for newsrooms and journalists, but a scan of the website may still be of interest to the general reader.[8]

And NewsGuard, a rapidly growing organization, draws on artificial intelligence to track and set "trust scores" for online information.[9] The company has journalistic roots, but it has tools and services for businesses that don't want to place advertisements on troublesome sites, for defense and national security organizations, for health care providers and organizations that want to make sure their patients are receiving accurate information—and for ordinary people who want to know more about what they are reading and what they can trust.

Other sites are not purely fact-checkers or literacy initiatives but are helpful for becoming a discerning consumer of health and medical news and a good detector of online nonsense. For instance, SciLine is an online resource from the American Association for the Advancement of Science that's designed for journalists. It has courses and it connects journalists and scientific experts, including in public health.[10] But some interviews and videos are available to the general public, for those who want to educate themselves a bit about the facts on public health, climate change, or other topics in the news. ScienceUpFirst (a Canadian organization) married science and social media savvy to address COVID-19.[11] Postpandemic, it has begun to post information on a range of public health and communication topics, including explaining how algorithms work. Similarly, an unusually broad health care alliance, called the Coalition for Trust in Health and Science, has set high goals to smash myths and restore trust in health care, but that too is still quite new and still taking form.[12] It hosts some myth-busting tools and resources on its website.

Keep Your Common Sense

The purveyors of fake news and disinformation manipulate us. They inflame our negative emotions, our anxieties and fears and resentments, so that when we encounter disinformation, it pushes our emotional buttons and overrides our common sense and caution.

It's up to us to stop, take a breath, and let our common sense, the slower and more thoughtful part of our brains, push back.

In other words, before you share, or repost, or just let loose online, slow down.

If you read something online and it sounds too good to be true, it could well be a mistake or a scam or a lie or some combination thereof. When you read something so terrifying that you feel an almost panicked obligation to share it as quickly and as widely as possible, that too is a time to slow down. That asteroid probably is not coming to destroy Earth in the next 48 hours (and even if it was, would your hasty post really stop it?). Before you share or disseminate, double-check. Is any reliable source reporting it? Or only some obscure internet site or social media personality that you've never heard of before (and may not actually exist). If you can't confirm information—whether heartening or terrifying—assume that it's probably false or at least distorted.

On health claims, confirm what you see online (or what your sister-in-law heard from her next-door neighbor's college roommate's ex-husband's mechanic) with a trusted health source. If you do not trust government agencies, try other sites that don't have a government overlay. The Mayo Clinic's online Health Library has clearly written and accessible information about symptoms, diseases, and other clinical problems.[13] Johns Hopkins Medicine also has a helpful guide to symptoms and diseases.[14] Most other health systems offer similar resources to the public (and some are multilingual).

A few acronyms and techniques might help. A librarian named Molly Beestrum developed the CRAP Test to evaluate websites. The acronym stands for currency/credibility, reliability, authority, and purpose/point of view. Those four categories prod you to ask questions such as: How recent is the information? Does the website include citations? What are the author's credentials? Does the author seem to be trying to push an agenda or sell you something?[15] Her road map is now commonly found as a resource on the websites of numerous college and university libraries. Similarly, a Washington State University digital literacy expert named Mike Caulfield came up with a model called SIFT. That stands for "Stop. Investigate the source. Find better coverage. Trace claims, quotes, and media to the original context."[16]

This isn't a comprehensive list. So when navigating the wonderful and terrible online landscape, remember: Learn. Confirm. Find your inner skeptic.

And One Last Thing

Subscribe to—and engage with—your local paper or to an innovative nonprofit trying to fill those news deserts and helping us stay safe, healthy, and informed.

NOTES

Introduction. Information Sick

1. Geoff Brumfiel and Meredith Rizzo, "Their Mom Died of COVID. They Say Conspiracy Theories Are What Really Killed Her," National Public Radio, April 24, 2022, https://www.npr.org/sections/health-shots/2022/04/24/1089786147/covid-conspiracy-theories.

2. "Nearly 108,000 Americans Died of Drug Overdoses in 2022, Breaking Record, CDC Says," CBS News, March 22, 2024, https://www.cbsnews.com/news/us-drug-overdose-deaths-2022-record/.

3. "Suicides in the U.S. Reached All-Time High in 2022, CDC Data Shows," Associated Press, August 10, 2023, https://www.nbcnews.com/health/mental-health/cdc-data-finds-suicides-reached-time-high-2022-rcna99327.

4. Latoya Hill and Samantha Artiga, "What Is Driving Widening Racial Disparities in Life Expectancy?," Kaiser Family Foundation, May 23, 2023, https://www.kff.org/racial-equity-and-health-policy/issue-brief/what-is-driving-widening-racial-disparities-in-life-expectancy/.

5. "Life Expectancy at Birth (Years)," World Health Organization, accessed April 21, 2024, https://www.who.int/data/gho/data/indicators/indicator-details/GHO/life-expectancy-at-birth-(years).

6. Hill and Artiga, "What Is Driving?"

7. "Heart Disease and African Americans," Office of Minority Health, US Department of Health and Human Services, 2023, https://minorityhealth.hhs.gov/heart-disease-and-african-americans.

8. Latoya Hill et al., "Key Data on Health and Health Care by Race and Ethnicity," Kaiser Family Foundation, March 15, 2023, https://www.kff.org/racial-equity-and-health-policy/report/key-data-on-health-and-health-care-by-race-and-ethnicity/.

9. "Suicide in Rural America," US Centers for Disease Control and Prevention, April 21, 2023, https://www.cdc.gov/ruralhealth/Suicide.html.

10. Brian Kennedy and Alec Tyson, "Americans' Trust in Scientists, Positive Views of Science Continue to Decline," Pew Research Center, November 14, 2023, https://www.pewresearch.org/science/2023/11/14/americans-trust-in-scientists-positive-views-of-science-continue-to-decline/.

11. Priya Chidambaram and Alice Burns, "Few Nursing Facility Residents and Staff Have Received the Latest COVID-19 Vaccine," Kaiser Family Foundation, February 13, 2024, https://www.kff.org/medicaid/issue-brief/few-nursing-facility-residents-and-staff-have-received-the-latest-covid-19-vaccine/.

12. Lena H. Sun, "CDC Data Shows Highest Level Yet of Vaccine Exemptions for Kindergartners," *Washington Post*, November 9, 2023, https://www.washingtonpost.com/health/2023/11/09/kindergarten-vaccine-exemptions-cdc-data/.

13. Elizabeth White, "Tragic Lee County Baby Death Linked to Vitamin K Shot Refusal," WRBL Columbus, February 13, 2024, https://news.yahoo.com/tragic-lee-county-baby-death-000556610.html.

14. Elia Ben-Ari, "Addressing the Challenges of Cancer Misinformation on Social Media," National Cancer Institute, September 9, 2021, https://www.cancer.gov/news-events/cancer-currents-blog/2021/cancer-misinformation-social-media.

15. Ellen McVay, "Social Media and Self-Diagnosis," Johns Hopkins Medicine, August 31, 2023, https://www.hopkinsmedicine.org/news/articles/2023/08/social-media-and-self-diagnosis.

16. Renee Garett and Sean D. Young, "The Role of Misinformation and Stigma in Opioid Use Disorder Treatment Uptake," *Substance Use and Misuse* 57, no. 8 (2022): 1332–36, https://doi.org/10.1080/10826084.2022.2079133.

17. "SciCheck," FactCheck.org, accessed February 4, 2025, Annenberg Public Policy Center, https://www.factcheck.org/scicheck/.

18. Brett Molina, "Facebook's Most Popular Article from January to March Was About Doctor Who Died After Getting COVID-19 Vaccine," *USA Today*, August 23, 2021, https://www.usatoday.com/story/tech/2021/08/23/facebook-content-transparency-report-most-popular-article/8239679002/.

19. Lydia Saad, "Historically Low Faith in U.S. Institutions Continues," Gallup, July 6, 2023, https://news.gallup.com/poll/508169/historically-low-faith-institutions-continues.aspx.

20. Jeff Bendix, "Which Health Care Professionals Are Leaving Their Jobs?," Medical Economics, October 26, 2023, https://www.medicaleconomics.com/view/which-health-care-professionals-are-leaving-their-jobs-.

21. Dan Diamond, "America Has a Life Expectancy Crisis. But It's Not a Political Priority," *Washington Post*, December 28, 2023, https://www.washingtonpost.com/health/2023/12/28/life-expectancy-no-political-response/.

22. Henry E. Brady and Thomas B. Kent, "Fifty Years of Declining Confidence and Increasing Polarization in Trust in American Institutions," *Daedalus* 151, no. 4 (2022): 43–66.

23. Saad, "Historically Low Faith."

24. Renée DiResta, *Invisible Rulers: The People Who Turn Lies into Reality* (PublicAffairs, 2024), 3.

25. "The Partisan Landscape and Views of the Parties," Pew Research Center, October 10, 2019, https://www.pewresearch.org/politics/2019/10/10/the-partisan-landscape-and-views-of-the-parties/.

26. Sara E. Gorman, *The Anatomy of Deception: Conspiracy Theories, Distrust, and Public Health in America* (Oxford University Press, 2024), 139.

27. Saher Kahn and Vignesh Ramachandran, "Millions Depend on Private Messaging Apps to Keep in Touch. They're Ripe with Misinformation," *PBS NewsHour*, November 5, 2021, https://www.pbs.org/newshour/world/millions-depend-on-private-messaging-apps-to-keep-in-touch-theyre-ripe-with-misinformation.

28. Benjamin Toff et al., *Avoiding the News: Reluctant Audiences for Journalism* (Columbia University Press, 2023).

Chapter 1. The Collapse of Local News

1. Eric Eyre, *Death in Mud Lick: A Coal Country Fight Against the Drug Companies That Delivered the Opioid Epidemic* (Scribner, 2020), 95–96.

2. Eyre, *Death in Mud Lick*. p. 95.

3. Lacie Pierson, "HD Media Closes Purchase of Charleston Gazette-Mail," *Charleston Gazette-Mail*, March 30, 2018, https://www.wvgazettemail.com/news/hd-media-closes-purchase-of-charleston-gazette-mail/article_dfd84f3b-a44e-5d6a-a30b-edfc068f2f8e.html.

4. Eric Eyre, classroom interview, April 6, 2022.

5. Eyre, classroom interview.

6. Knight Foundation, *American Views 2022: Part 2, Trust Media and Democracy* (Knight Foundation and Gallup, 2023).

7. Penelope Muse Abernathy, "The State of Local News," Local News Initiative, November 16, 2023, https://localnewsinitiative.northwestern.edu/projects/state-of-local-news/2023/report/.

8. Abernathy, "State of Local News."

9. Abernathy, "State of Local News."

10. Mason Walker, "U.S. Newsroom Employment Has Fallen 26% Since 2008," Pew Research Center, July 13, 2021, https://www.pewresearch.org/short-reads/2021/07/13/u-s-newsroom-employment-has-fallen-26-since-2008/.

11. Alexandra Bruell, "Your Local Newspaper Might Not Have a Single Reporter," *Wall Street Journal*, November 24, 2023, https://www.wsj.com/business/media/your-local-newspaper-might-not-have-a-single-reporter-f62b803d.

12. Taylor Telford, "Warren Buffett Said Newspapers Were Going to Disappear. Now They've Disappeared from His Portfolio," *Washington Post*, January 29, 2020, https://www.washingtonpost.com/business/2020/01/29/warren-buffett-said-newspapers-were-going-disappear-now-hes-disappearing-industry/.

13. Leonard Downie Jr. and Michael Schudson, "The Reconstruction of American Journalism," *Columbia Journalism Review*, November 2009, https://

archives.cjr.org/reconstruction/the_reconstruction_of_american.php (emphasis in the original).

14. Eileen Buckley, "Judge Orders Hospital to Treat COVID Patient with Experimental Drug," WKBW Buffalo, January 18, 2021, https://www.wkbw.com/news/coronavirus/judge-orders-hospital-to-treat-covid-patient-with-experimental-drug.

15. Carolyn T. Bramante et al., "Randomized Trial of Metformin, Ivermectin, and Fluvoxamine for Covid-19," *New England Journal of Medicine* 387, no. 7 (2022): 599–610, https://doi.org/10.1056/NEJMoa2201662.

16. Mike Argento, "Ivermectin: Wife of York County Man on 'Death's Doorstep' from COVID Sues UPMC to Use Drug," *York Daily Record*, December 1, 2021, https://www.ydr.com/story/news/2021/12/01/lawsuit-aims-force-upmc-hospital-treat-man-covid-ivermectin-york-county-pa/8812207002/.

17. Mike Argento, "Man Whose Wife Won a Court Battle to Treat His COVID-19 with Ivermectin Has Died," *York Daily Record*, December 13, 2021, https://www.ydr.com/story/news/2021/12/13/pa-man-who-won-court-battle-treat-his-covid-ivermectin-has-died/6493657001/.

18. Margaret Sullivan, *Ghosting the News: Local Journalism and the Crisis of American Democracy* (Columbia Global Reports, 2020).

19. "Where's the Urgency?," editorial, *Baltimore Sun*, January 26, 2009.

20. B'more for Healthy Babies, home page, accessed April 11, 2024, http://healthybabiesbaltimore.com.

21. Cody Boteler et al., "New Baltimore Sun Owner Insults Staff in Meeting, Says Paper Should Mimic Fox45," *Baltimore Banner*, January 17, 2024, https://www.thebaltimorebanner.com/economy/baltimore-sun-david-smith-sinclair-owner-F77S3D47ORD7LNEPZ7PJCXSLWM/.

22. Andrea K. McDaniels, classroom interview, April 6, 2022.

23. McDaniels, classroom interview.

24. McKay Coppins, "Alden Global Capital, the Hedge Fund Killing Newspapers," *Atlantic*, October 14, 2023, https://www.theatlantic.com/magazine/archive/2021/11/alden-global-capital-killing-americas-newspapers/620171/.

25. Peter Kendall, in discussion with Joanne Kenen, March 15, 2024.

26. Kendall, in discussion with Kenen.

27. Michael Ewens et al., "Local Journalism Under Private Equity Ownership," NBER Working Paper 29743 (National Bureau of Economic Research, February 2022), https://doi.org/10.3386/w29743.

28. Ewens et al., "Local Journalism," abstract.

29. Shraddha Chakradhar, "'An Immediate Drop in Content': A New Study Shows What Happens When Big Companies Take over Local News," Nieman Lab, April 20, 2022, https://www.niemanlab.org/2022/04/an-immediate-drop-in-content-a-new-study-shows-what-happens-when-big-companies-take-over-local-news/.

30. Naomi Forman-Katz, "For National Radio Day, Key Facts About Radio Listeners and the Radio Industry in the U.S.," Pew Research Center, August 17, 2023, https://www.pewresearch.org/short-reads/2023/08/17/for-national-radio-day-key-facts-about-radio-listeners-and-the-radio-industry-in-the-us/.

31. Robert Lang, classroom interview, April 6, 2022.

32. Lang, classroom interview.

33. Lang, classroom interview.

34. Salem News Channel, home page, accessed February 6, 2025, http://salemnewschannel.com.

35. Ted Johnson, "Air America Folds," *Variety*, January 21, 2010, https://variety.com/2010/biz/opinion/air-america-folds-39694/.

36. Paul Farhi, "What Wendy Rieger Learned from Washington," *Washington Post*, December 27, 2021, https://www.washingtonpost.com/lifestyle/media/wendy-rieger-retires/2021/12/26/b0961cfe-627f-11ec-8ce3-9454d0b46d42_story.html.

37. "Investor Relations," Sinclair, accessed October 25, 2023, https://sbgi.net/investor-relations/.

38. Angela Chen, in discussion with Joanne Kenen, November 16, 2023.

39. Chen, in discussion with Kenen.

40. Gregory J. Martin and Joshua McCrain, "Local News and National Politics," *American Political Science Review* 113, no. 2 (2019): 372–84, https://doi.org/10.1017/s0003055418000965.

41. Sarah E. Gollust et al., "Television News Coverage of Public Health Issues and Implications for Public Health Policy," *Annual Reviews* 40 (April 2019): 167–85, https://doi.org/10.1146/annurev-publhealth-040218-044017.

42. Gollust et al., "Television News Coverage."

43. Josef Verbanac and Claire Golding, eds., "Pink Slime: Fake-Local News," Iffy.news, accessed November 6, 2022, https://iffy.news/pink-slime-fake-local-news/.

44. Sara Rafsky, "Tow Center Audience Study: Reader Perspectives on Partisan Local News Sites," *Columbia Journalism Review*, September 19, 2022, https://www.cjr.org/tow_center_reports/tow-center-audience-study-reader-perspectives-on-local-partisan-news-sites.php.

45. Priyanjana Bengani, "Hundreds of 'Pink Slime' Local News Outlets Are Distributing Algorithmic Stories and Conservative Talking Points," *Columbia Journalism Review*, December 18, 2019, https://www.cjr.org/tow_center_reports/hundreds-of-pink-slime-local-news-outlets-are-distributing-algorithmic-stories-conservative-talking-points.php; Priyanjana Bengani, "The Metric Media Network Runs More Than 1,200 Local News Sites. Here Are Some of the Non-Profits Funding Them," *Columbia Journalism Review*, October 14, 2021, https://www.cjr.org/tow_center_reports/metric-media-lobbyists-funding.php; Priyanjana Bengani, "'Pink Slime' Network Gets $1.6M Election Boost from PACs Backed by Oil-and-Gas, Shipping Magnates," *Columbia Journalism Review*, October 31, 2022, https://www.cjr.org/tow_center/pink-slime-network-gets-1-6m-election-boost

-from-pacs-backed-by-oil-and-gas-shipping-magnates.php; Asa Royal and Philip M. Napoli, *Local Journalism's Possible Future: Metric Media and Its Approach to Community Information Needs* (DeWitt Wallace Center for Media and Democracy, July 2021), https://dewitt.sanford.duke.edu/wp-content/uploads/sites/3/2021/07/Future-of-Local-News.pdf.

46. Priyanjana Bengani, "The Nonprofits and PACS That Spent $14 Million on the Metric Media Network in 2021–22," *Columbia Journalism Review*, August 8, 2024, https://www.cjr.org/tow_center/the-non-profits-and-pacs-that-spent-14-million-on-the-metric-media-network-in-2021-22.php.

47. Anna Massoglia, "'Dark Money' Networks Hide Political Agendas Behind Fake News Sites," OpenSecrets News, May 22, 2020, https://www.opensecrets.org/news/2020/05/dark-money-networks-fake-news-sites/.

48. Steven Brill, "The New Pink Slime Media," Semafor, June 2, 2024, https://www.semafor.com/article/06/02/2024/the-new-pink-slime-media; Jem Bartholomew, "The Rise and Rise of Partisan Local Newsrooms," *Columbia Journalism Review*, September 19, 2022, https://www.cjr.org/tow_center/the-rise-of-partisan-local-newsrooms.php.

49. The Virality Project, *Memes, Magnets and Microchips: Narrative Dynamics Around COVID-19 Vaccines* (2022), Stanford Digital Repository, https://doi.org/10.25740/mx395xj8490.

50. *Apopka Times*, home page, archived April 12, 2022, at https://web.archive.org/web/20220412000939/https://apopkatimes.com/.

51. Marianne Todd, "Conservative Media Network Behind Mystery Paper in New Mexico Mailboxes," *Santa Fe New Mexican*, November 18, 2022, https://www.santafenewmexican.com/news/local_news/conservative-media-network-behind-mystery-paper-in-new-mexico-mailboxes/article_8aeb756a-6564-11ed-906f-0b4562328d38.html; Josh Kelety, "Partisan Mailer Poses as Catholic Newspaper in Arizona," AP News, November 4, 2022, https://apnews.com/article/2022-midterm-elections-religion-arizona-phoenix-newspapers-a86b9055979e785bfe5af76cfb4def32.

52. Sarah Blaskey, "Powerbrokers: How FPL Secretly Took Over a Florida News Site and Used It to Bash Critics," *Miami Herald*, July 25, 2022, https://www.miamiherald.com/news/politics-government/state-politics/article263757423.html.

53. David Folkenflik et al., "In the Southeast, Power Company Money Flows to News Sites That Attack Their Critics," NPR, December 19, 2022, https://www.npr.org/2022/12/19/1143753129/power-companies-florida-alabama-media-investigation-consulting-firm.

54. Elizabeth Weise, "Hackers Use Typosquatting to Dupe the Unwary with Fake News, Sites," *USA Today*, December 1, 2016, https://www.usatoday.com/story/tech/news/2016/12/01/hackers-use-typo-squatting-lure-unwary-url-hijacking/94683460/.

55. Sam Brodey, "Will Kyrsten Sinema's 'Self-Destructive' Moves Take Her Down?," *Daily Beast*, August 12, 2022, https://www.thedailybeast.com/will-kyrsten-sinemas-self-destructive-moves-take-her-down.

56. Philadelphia Center for Gun Violence Reporting, home page, accessed April 11, 2024, http://www.pcgvr.org.

57. "CARE Act—California Health and Human Services," California Health and Human Services Agency, accessed December 15, 2023, https://www.chhs.ca.gov/care-act/; Jocelyn Wiener, "Gavin Newsom Signs Law in 'Overhaul' of Mental Health System. It Changes Decades of Practice," CalMatters, October 10, 2023, https://calmatters.org/health/2023/10/california-mental-health-involuntary-treatment-law/.

58. Linda Mimms (vice chair, Schizophrenia and Psychosis Action Alliance), in discussion with Joanne Kenen, October 10, 2023.

59. Saja Hindi, "Abortion Rights Activists in Colorado Look to State Constitution to Secure Access," *Boulder (CO) Daily Camera*, October 3, 2023, https://www.dailycamera.com/2023/10/03/colorado-abortion-pill-reversal-2024-ballot/.

60. Thomas Garrett, "It's All About the Vape," *Baxter Bulletin* (AR), February 11, 2015, https://www.proquest.com/newspapers/all-about-vape/docview/1673095666/se-2.

61. Sarah E. Gollust et al., "Local Television News Coverage of the Affordable Care Act: Emphasizing Politics over Consumer Information," *American Journal of Public Health* 107, no. 5 (2017): 687–93, https://doi.org/10.2105/ajph.2017.303659.

62. Gollust et al., "Local Television News Coverage."

63. Debbie Bryce, "Insurance Agents Frustrated by U.S. Health Law," *Idaho State Journal*, October 20, 2013, https://www.idahostatejournal.com/members/insurance-agents-frustrated-by-u-s-health-law/article_1d713a2e-3959-11e3-8156-0019bb2963f4.html.

64. Trudy Lieberman, "Navigating the Labyrinth: A Primer on Obamacare Enrollment for Health Reporters," *Columbia Journalism Review*, November 3, 2017, https://www.cjr.org/covering_the_health_care_fight/obamacare-enrollment-subsidies.php.

65. Munira Z. Gunja and Sara R. Collins, "Who Are the Remaining Uninsured and Why Do They Lack Coverage?," issue brief, Commonwealth Fund, August 28, 2019, https://www.commonwealthfund.org/publications/issue-briefs/2019/aug/who-are-remaining-uninsured-and-why-do-they-lack-coverage.

66. Sarah Fioroni, "Local News Most Trusted in Keeping Americans Informed About Their Communities," Knight Foundation, May 19, 2022, https://knightfoundation.org/articles/local-news-most-trusted-in-keeping-americans-informed-about-their-communities/.

67. "Orthodontist Calls on Voters to Keep Fluoride," *Box Elder News Journal* (Brigham City, UT), October 11, 2023, https://www.benewsjournal.com/articles/orthodontist-calls-on-voters-to-keep-fluoride/.

68. Robert S. Eshelman, "The Danger of Fair and Balanced," *Columbia Journalism Review*, May 1, 2014, https://archives.cjr.org/essay/the_danger_of_fair_and_balance.php.

69. Gretchen Sisson et al., "'The Stakes Are So High': Interviews with Progressive Journalists Reporting on Abortion," *Contraception* 96, no. 6 (2017): 395–400, https://doi.org/10.1016/j.contraception.2017.08.005.

70. Hannah Fingerhut et al., "An Iowa Meteorologist Started Talking About Climate Change on Newscasts. Then Came the Harassment," AP News, July 8, 2023, https://apnews.com/article/meteorologist-harassment-threats-climate-change-iowa-bf91adbd26ca5e97507406947b47d684.

71. Hoag Levins, "Vaccine Scientist Slams Media for False Balance," *LDI Health Economist*, April 2014, http://ldihealtheconomist.com/he000096.shtml.

72. Levins, "Vaccine Scientist Slams Media."

73. Nick Robins-Early, "How Anti-Vaxxers and Ivermectin Advocates Have Co-Opted US Local News," *Guardian*, November 30, 2021, https://www.theguardian.com/media/2021/nov/03/how-anti-vaxxers-and-ivermectin-advocates-have-co-opted-local-news.

74. Jerome Adams, "Lunch Talk: Dr. Jerome Adams, Former Surgeon General of the U.S.," in discussion with Kelsey Ryan, Health Journalism 2023, Association of Health Care Journalists conference, St. Louis, MO, March 11, 2023.

75. Angie Moreschi and Larry Deal, "Lack of Transparency Concerns over Billions in Opioid Settlement Money Distributions," NBC Montana, October 17, 2023, https://nbcmontana.com/news/spotlight-on-america/lack-of-transparency-concerns-over-billions-in-opioid-settlement-money-distributions.

76. J. David McSwane, "'Pain and Profit' Investigation Spurs Sweeping Bipartisan Fix for Texas' Medicaid Managed-Care Mess," *Dallas News*, February 25, 2019, https://www.dallasnews.com/news/politics/2019/02/25/pain-profit-investigation-spurs-sweeping-bipartisan-fix-for-texas-medicaid-managed-care-mess/.

77. J. David McSwane, "Pain and Profit: Texas Health Agency Beefs Up Oversight of Medicaid Companies as House Inquiry Begins," *Dallas News*, August 26, 2018, https://www.dallasnews.com/news/2018/08/26/pain-profit-texas-health-agency-beefs-up-oversight-of-medicaid-companies-as-house-inquiry-begins/.

78. Julie A. Ward et al., "Pandemic-Related Workplace Violence and Its Impact on Public Health Officials, March 2020–January 2021," *American Journal of Public Health* 112, no. 5 (2022): 736–46, https://doi.org/10.2105/ajph.2021.306649.

79. Anna Gustafson, "Berrien Co. Health Officials Resign, Citing 'Politicization of Public Health' During Pandemic," *Michigan Advance*, October 19, 2021, https://michiganadvance.com/2021/10/19/berrien-co-health-officials-resign-citing-politicization-of-public-health-during-pandemic/.

80. Nadia Kounang, "The Pandemic Has Pushed More Than 250 Public Health Officials out the Door," CNN, May 23, 2021, https://www.cnn.com/2021/05/23/health/public-health-officials-quit/index.html.

81. Audrey Dutton, "'It Should Be Stopped': Idaho Medical Group Files Complaint Against Dr. Ryan Cole," *Idaho Capital Sun*, October 11, 2021, https://idahocapitalsun.com/2021/10/11/it-should-be-stopped-idaho-medical-group-files-complaint-against-dr-ryan-cole/.

82. Mike Baker and Danielle Ivory, "Why Public Health Faces a Crisis Across the U.S.," *New York Times*, October 18, 2021, https://www.nytimes.com/2021/10/18/us/coronavirus-public-health.html.

83. National Trust for Local News, home page, accessed December 15, 2023, https://www.nationaltrustforlocalnews.org/.

84. Press Forward, home page, accessed December 15, 2023, https://www.pressforward.news/.

85. "About Us," Report for America, accessed December 15, 2023, https://www.reportforamerica.org/about-us/.

86. "About the Mental Health Project," *Seattle Times*, September 14, 2023, https://www.seattletimes.com/seattle-news/mental-health/about-the-mental-health-project/.

87. Hannah Furfaro, classroom interview, November 7, 2022.

88. Furfaro, classroom interview.

89. Hannah Furfaro, "Inside Seattle Children's, Staff Increasingly Restraining Kids in Crisis," *Seattle Times*, December 23, 2023, https://www.seattletimes.com/seattle-news/mental-health/inside-seattle-childrens-staff-increasingly-restraining-kids-in-crisis/.

90. Furfaro, classroom interview.

91. Hannah Furfaro, "WA Kids Are Stuck in Hospitals. State Lawmakers Want One Person to Take Charge," *Seattle Times*, April 12, 2023, https://www.seattletimes.com/seattle-news/mental-health/lawmakers-pass-bill-to-change-how-wa-cares-for-youth-stuck-in-hospitals/.

92. Autumn Phillips, "How the Post and Courier Raised More Than $1 Million for a South Carolina-Wide Investigative Fund and Education Lab," Better News, September 2021, https://betternews.org/how-the-post-and-courier-raised-more-than-1-million-to-support-its-journalism/.

93. Tony Bartelme, in discussion with Joanne Kenen, September 21, 2023.

94. Bartelme, in discussion with Kenen.

95. "About Uncovered," *Post and Courier*, accessed February 6, 2025, http://postandcourier.com/uncovered.

96. Tony Bartelme et al., "News Deserts and Weak Ethics Laws Allow Corruption to Run Rampant in SC," *Post and Courier*, February 13, 2021, https://www.postandcourier.com/uncovered/news-deserts-and-weak-ethics-laws-allow-corruption-to-run-rampant-in-sc/article_df3f64fe-5a63-11eb-aa62-4fb6abe764b6.html. All of the projects cited can be found on the "Uncovered" home page, accessed February 6, 2025, http://postandcourier.com/uncovered. They are generally free, no subscription required.

97. Andrew Brown, "Golf, Beaches and Power: How Utilities Wine and Dine the Public Officials That Set Your Rates," *Post and Courier*, December 28, 2022, https://www.postandcourier.com/business/golf-beaches-and-power-how-utilities-wine-and-dine-the-public-officials-that-set-your/article_69a1a33c-ea55-11e7-ac03-bbac632ad01b.html.

98. Stephen Hobbs and Thad Moore, "SC Superintendent Lived Rent-Free in Townhouse Meant for Teacher Recruitment," *Post and Courier*, August 7, 2021, https://www.postandcourier.com/uncovered/sc-superintendent-lived-rent-free-in-townhouse-meant-for-teacher-recruitment/article_8d903620-ee14-11eb-9074-5bbcba0ba8a9.html; Avery G. Wilks and Joseph Cranney, "South Carolina Politicians Blow Off Their Ethics Fines with Few Consequences," *Post and Courier*, August 14, 2021, https://www.postandcourier.com/uncovered/south-carolina-politicians-blow-off-their-ethics-fines-with-few-consequences/article_dff3d734-f90c-11eb-b224-f31c3af0e987.html.

99. Tony Bartelme, "A South Carolina Sheriff. A Rape Claim. And Silence from SLED," *Post and Courier*, January 22, 2022, https://www.postandcourier.com/uncovered/a-south-carolina-sheriff-a-rape-claim-and-silence-from-sled/article_fd0b409a-731a-11ec-84f9-271c0469a9dd.html; Kailey Cota, "MOLD U: Hundreds of Students Struggle with Mold in Campus Dorms, USC System Unfit to Analyze Reports," *Post and Courier*, October 29, 2022, https://www.postandcourier.com/uncovered/mold-u-hundreds-of-students-struggle-with-mold-in-campus-dorms-usc-system-unfit-to/article_422998de-555b-11ed-a451-876dc9b216ba.html; Tony Bartelme, "SC Coroner Flouts Transparency Laws, Hires Ex-SC State Police Chief Caught in Scam," *Post and Courier*, December 18, 2022, https://www.postandcourier.com/news/sc-coroner-flouts-transparency-laws-hires-ex-sc-state-police-chief-caught-in-scam/article_16598098-71b2-11ed-9e6a-2f49d091c96b.html.

100. Stephen Hobbs et al., "As SC Town Struggles with Water Issues, Residents Wonder Why Councilman Didn't Warn Them," *Post and Courier*, June 26, 2021, https://www.postandcourier.com/uncovered/as-sc-town-struggles-with-water-issues-residents-wonder-why-councilman-didnt-warn-them/article_7b277c42-b1af-11eb-ad4e-c38b007837ca.html.

101. Bartelme, in discussion with Kenen.

102. "Rising Waters: Climate Stories of the South," *Post and Courier*, accessed December 15, 2023, https://www.postandcourier.com/rising-waters/.

103. Tony Bartelme, "Competition or Collaboration: Tony Bartelme on News Deserts," American Association for the Advancement of Science, April 13, 2021, https://www.aaas.org/news/competition-or-collaboration-tony-bartelme-news-deserts.

104. Bartelme, "Competition or Collaboration."

105. Bartelme, "Competition or Collaboration."

106. Bartelme, in discussion with Kenen.

Chapter 2. The Fracturing of National News

1. Ricardo Alonso-Zaldivar (retired journalist), in discussion with Joanne Kenen, August 28, 2023.
2. Alonso-Zaldivar, in discussion with Kenen.
3. Alonso-Zaldivar, in discussion with Kenen.
4. Alonso-Zaldivar, in discussion with Kenen.
5. Alonso-Zaldivar, in discussion with Kenen.
6. Alonso-Zaldivar, in discussion with Kenen.
7. Jay Rosen (@jayrosen_nyu), "Not the odds, but the stakes. That's my shorthand for the organizing principle we most need in journalists covering the 2024 campaign. Not who has what chances of winning, but the consequences for American democracy. Not the odds, but the stakes," X, March 7, 2023, https://twitter.com/jayrosen_nyu/status/1633169838175649795.
8. Dan Froomkin, "*The Washington Post* Has a Bezos Problem," *Columbia Journalism Review*, September 27, 2022, https://www.cjr.org/special_report/washington-post-jeff-bezos.php.
9. Filipe R. Campante and Daniel Hojman, "Media and Polarization: Evidence from the Introduction of Broadcast TV in the United States," *Journal of Public Economics* 100 (April 2013): 79–92, https://doi.org/10.1016/j.jpubeco.2013.02.006.
10. Campante and Hojman, "Media and Polarization."
11. James Gattuso, "Back to Muzak? Congress and the Un-Fairness Doctrine," Heritage Foundation, May 23, 2007, https://www.heritage.org/government-regulation/report/back-muzak-congress-and-the-un-fairness-doctrine.
12. "Health Coverage in the US Media," Pew Research Center, November 24, 2008, https://www.pewresearch.org/journalism/2008/11/24/health-news-coverage-in-the-u-s-media/.
13. Andrew Tyndall, "It Is Remarkable How Little Attention Has Been Paid to Issues Coverage During This Presidential Cycle," *Tyndall Report*, October 25, 2016, http://tyndallreport.com/comment/20/5778.
14. Thomas Patterson, "News Coverage of the 2016 Presidential Primaries: Horse Race Reporting Has Consequences," Harvard Kennedy School, December 2016, https://www.hks.harvard.edu/publications/news-coverage-2016-presidential-primaries-horse-race-reporting-has-consequences.
15. "Research: Media Coverage of the 2016 Election," Shorenstein Center on Media, Politics and Public Policy, September 7, 2016, https://shorensteincenter.org/research-media-coverage-2016-election/.
16. Thomas E. Patterson, "A Tale of Two Elections: CBS and Fox News' Portrayal of the 2020 Presidential Campaign," Shorenstein Center on Media, Politics and Public Policy, December 17, 2020, https://shorensteincenter.org/patterson-2020-election-coverage/.
17. Paul Bond, "Leslie Moonves on Donald Trump: 'It May Not Be Good for America, but It's Damn Good for CBS,'" *Hollywood Reporter*, February 29, 2016,

https://www.hollywoodreporter.com/news/general-news/leslie-moonves-donald-trump-may-871464/.

18. Alex Weprin, "CBS CEO Les Moonves Clarifies Donald Trump 'Good for CBS' Comment," *Politico*, October 19, 2016, https://www.politico.com/blogs/on-media/2016/10/cbs-ceo-les-moonves-clarifies-donald-trump-good-for-cbs-comment-229996.

19. Emily Stewart, "Donald Trump Rode $5 Billion in Free Media to the White House," *The Street*, November 20, 2016, https://www.thestreet.com/politics/donald-trump-rode-5-billion-in-free-media-to-the-white-house-13896916.

20. Jim Morrill, "Covering the 2020 Election: Horse Race or Citizens Agenda?," Nieman Reports, January 24, 2019, https://niemanreports.org/articles/covering-the-2020-election-horserace-or-citizens-agenda/.

21. There's a fair amount of consumer health reporting on cable, such as information about new "breakthroughs" and trends, but not sustained coverage of knotty policy.

22. Chris Stirewalt, *Broken News: Why the Media Rage Machine Divides America and How to Fight Back* (Center Street, 2022), 7.

23. Alex Paterson, "Fox News Has Aired 86 Segments About Trans People Since President Biden Took Office," Media Matters for America, March 22, 2021, https://www.mediamatters.org/fox-news/fox-news-has-aired-86-segments-about-trans-people-president-biden-took-office.

24. Dannagal Goldthwaite Young, *Wrong: How Media, Politics, and Identity Drive Our Appetite for Misinformation* (Johns Hopkins University Press, 2023).

25. "Cable News Fact Sheet," Pew Research Center, September 14, 2023, https://www.pewresearch.org/journalism/fact-sheet/cable-news/.

26. Andrey Simonov et al., "The Persuasive Effect of Fox News: Non-Compliance with Social Distancing During the Covid-19 Pandemic," NBER Working Paper 27237 (National Bureau of Economic Research, May 2020, revised July 2020), https://doi.org/10.3386/w27237.

27. Simonov et al., "Persuasive Effect of Fox News," 7.

28. Stirewalt, *Broken News*, 7.

29. Kevin Reuning and Nick Dietrich, "Media Coverage, Public Interest, and Support in the 2016 Republican Invisible Primary," *Perspectives on Politics* 17, no. 2 (2018): 326–39, https://doi.org/10.1017/s1537592718003274.

30. Adam J. Berinsky and Michele F. Margolis, "Missing Voices: Polling and Health Care," *Journal of Health Politics Policy and Law* 36, no. 6 (2011): 975. https://doi.org/10.1215/03616878-1460551.

31. Richard Besser, classroom interview, May 18, 2022.

32. Besser, classroom interview.

33. Besser, classroom interview.

34. Jerome Adams, "Lunch Talk: Dr. Jerome Adams, Former Surgeon General of the U.S.," in discussion with Kelsey Ryan, Health Journalism 2023, Association of Health Care Journalists conference, St. Louis, MO, March 11, 2023.

35. Adams, "Lunch Talk."

36. Patterson, "News Coverage of the 2016 Presidential Primaries."

37. Patterson, "News Coverage of the 2016 Presidential Primaries."

38. Jay Rosen, "It's Time for the Media to Choose: Neutrality or Democracy?," interview by Nicole Hemmer, *The Ezra Klein Show* (podcast), *New York Times*, November 12, 2021, https://www.nytimes.com/2021/11/12/podcasts/transcript-ezra-klein-show-jay-rosen.html.

39. Lena H. Sun et al., "Doctors Who Put Lives at Risk with Covid Misinformation Rarely Punished," *Washington Post*, July 26, 2023, https://www.washingtonpost.com/health/2023/07/26/covid-misinformation-doctor-discipline/.

40. Apoorva Mandavilli, "Why We're Still Breathing Dirty Indoor Air," *New York Times*, December 11, 2023, https://www.nytimes.com/2023/11/20/health/indoor-air-covid-pollution.html.

41. Dan Diamond, "Trump Officials Interfered with CDC Reports on Covid-19," *Politico*, September 12, 2020, https://www.politico.com/news/2020/09/11/exclusive-trump-officials-interfered-with-cdc-reports-on-covid-19-412809.

42. John Carreyrou, "Hot Startup Theranos Has Struggled with Its Blood-Test Technology," *Wall Street Journal*, October 16, 2015, https://www.wsj.com/articles/theranos-has-struggled-with-blood-tests-1444881901.

43. Amy Goldstein, *Janesville: An American Story* (Simon and Schuster, 2017).

44. Amy Goldstein, classroom interview, November 14, 2022.

45. Goldstein, classroom interview.

46. Goldstein, classroom interview.

47. Rosen, "It's Time for the Media to Choose."

48. Benjamin Toff et al., *Avoiding the News: Reluctant Audiences for Journalism* (Columbia University Press, 2024).

49. Besser, classroom interview.

50. Celine Gounder (senior fellow and editor-at-large, KFF Health News), in discussion with Joanne Kenen, November 27, 2023.

51. Gounder, in discussion with Kenen.

52. Gounder, in discussion with Kenen.

53. David Folkenflik, "With Layoffs, NPR Becomes Latest Media Outlet to Cut Jobs," NPR, February 23, 2023, https://www.npr.org/2023/02/22/1158710498/npr-layoffs-2023.

54. Margot Sanger-Katz, classroom interview, November 14, 2022.

55. Sanger-Katz, classroom interview.

56. Sanger-Katz, classroom interview.

57. Matt Giles, "When Richard Nixon Declared War on the Media," Longreads, November 8, 2018, https://longreads.com/2018/11/08/when-richard-nixon-declared-war-on-the-media/.

58. Corky Siemaszko, "Oklahoma County Leaders Caught on Audio Talking About Killing Reporters and Complaining They Can No Longer Lynch Black

People," NBC News, April 17, 2023, https://www.nbcnews.com/news/us-news
/oklahoma-county-leaders-caught-audio-talking-killing-reporters-complai
-rcna80055.

59. Chris Walker, "Trump Proposes Imprisoning Journalists Who Don't Name Sources," Truthout, October 24, 2022, https://truthout.org/articles/trump-pro poses-imprisoning-journalists-who-dont-name-sources/; Nina Golgowski, "Trump Warns Critical News Media 'Will Pay a Big Price' If He's Reelected," *Huffington Post*, September 25, 2023, https://www.huffpost.com/entry/trump-threatens-news -media-critical-of-him_n_651189ffe4b088d5608c6c94.

60. Brian Stelter, "White House Pulls CNN Reporter Jim Acosta's Pass After Contentious News Conference," CNN, November 7, 2018, https://www.cnn.com /2018/11/07/media/trump-cnn-press-conference/index.html.

61. John Cassidy, "'Sharpiegate' and Donald Trump's Perpetual Cone of Uncertainty," *New Yorker*, September 6, 2019, https://www.newyorker.com/news/our -columnists/sharpiegate-and-donald-trumps-perpetual-cone-of-uncertainty.

62. Lesley Stahl, "Deadline Club Awards 2018 Dinner Conversation with Judy Woodruff and Lesley Stahl," in discussion with Judy Woodruff, Deadline Club Awards 2018, New York City, May 21, 2018, posted May 22, 2018, by Deadline Club, YouTube, 31 min., 3 sec., https://www.youtube.com/watch?v=nq6Tt--uAfs.

63. Megan Brenan, "Americans' Trust in Media Remains Near Record Low," Gallup, October 18, 2022, https://news.gallup.com/poll/403166/americans-trust -media-remains-near-record-low.aspx.

64. Daniel Hopkins and Tori Gorton, "Unsubscribed and Undemanding: Partisanship and the Minimal Effects of a Field Experiment Encouraging Local News Consumption," *American Journal of Political Science*, ahead of print, March 19, 2024, https://doi.org/10.1111/ajps.12845.

Chapter 3. The Flood of Misinformation

1. Brandy Zadrozny, host, *Truthers: Tiffany Dover Is Dead*, podcast, season 1, episode 3, "Who Does That?," NBC News, April 25, 2022, https://podcasts.apple .com/us/podcast/who-does-that/id1618512442?i=1000558584581.

2. Brandy Zadrozny, host, *Truthers: Tiffany Dover Is Dead*, podcast, season 1, episode 1, "Needle In," NBC News, April 18, 2022, https://podcasts.apple.com/us /podcast/needle-in/id1618512442?i=1000557899441.

3. Zadrozny, "Needle In."

4. Brandy Zadrozny, classroom interview, April 22, 2022.

5. Brandy Zadrozny, host, *Truthers: Tiffany Dover Is Dead*, podcast, season 1, episode 5, "Tiffany Dover Is Alive," NBC News, May 9, 2022, https://podcasts.apple .com/us/podcast/tiffany-dover-is-alive/id1618512442?i=1000560028041.

6. Zadrozny, "Needle In."

7. Brandy Zadrozny, host, *Truthers: Tiffany Dover Is Dead*, podcast, season 1, episode 6, "Special Episode: Tiffany Dover Speaks," NBC News, April 10, 2023,

https://podcasts.apple.com/us/podcast/special-episode-tiffany-dover-speaks/id1618512442?i=1000608157057.

8. Irene Pasquetto and Jennifer Nilsen, "The Abortion-Breast Cancer Myth: A Cloaked Science Case Study," Media Manipulation Casebook, May 17, 2021, https://mediamanipulation.org/case-studies/abortion-breast-cancer-myth-cloaked-science-case-study. The claims about abortion and breast cancer are an enduring myth that has its roots in a single low-quality Japanese study done in the 1950s.

9. US Congress, House, Committee on Government Reform, *Comprehensive Medical Care for Bioterrorism Exposure—Are We Making Evidenced-Based Decisions? What Are the Research Needs? Hearing Before the Committee on Government Reform*, 107th Cong., 1st sess., 2001, https://www.govinfo.gov/content/pkg/CHRG-107hhrg77497/html/CHRG-107hhrg77497.htm.

10. Vanessa Boudewyns et al., "Awareness of Misinformation in Health-Related Advertising," in *Misinformation and Mass Audiences*, ed. Brian G. Southwell et al. (University of Texas Press, 2018), 38.

11. Soroush Vosoughi et al., "The Spread of True and False News Online," *Science* 359, no. 6380 (2018): 1146–51, https://doi.org/10.1126/science.aap9559.

12. Vosoughi et al., "The Spread of True and False News Online," 1146.

13. Renée DiResta, *Invisible Rulers: The People Who Turn Lies into Reality* (PublicAffairs, 2024).

14. Richard Bruns et al., "COVID-19 Vaccine Misinformation and Disinformation Costs an Estimated $50 to $300 Million Each Day," Johns Hopkins Center for Health Security, October 20, 2021, https://centerforhealthsecurity.org/sites/default/files/2023-02/20211020-misinformation-disinformation-cost.pdf.

15. "Infodemic," World Health Organization, accessed October 10, 2023, https://www.who.int/health-topics/infodemic#tab=tab_1.

16. Sophia A. Rosenfeld, *Democracy and Truth: A Short History* (University of Pennsylvania Press, 2018), 173–74.

17. Elizabeth A. Gage-Bouchard et al., "Is Cancer Information Exchanged on Social Media Scientifically Accurate?," *Journal of Cancer Education* 33, no. 6 (2018): 1328–32, https://doi.org/10.1007/s13187-017-1254-z.

18. Jieun Shin et al., "The Diffusion of Misinformation on Social Media: Temporal Pattern, Message, and Source," *Computers in Human Behavior* 83 (June 2018): 278–87, https://doi.org/10.1016/j.chb.2018.02.008.

19. "Tracking AI-Enabled Misinformation: 802 'Unreliable AI-Generated News' Websites (and Counting), Plus the Top False Narratives Generated by Artificial Intelligence Tools," NewsGuard, April 15, 2024, https://www.newsguardtech.com/special-reports/ai-tracking-center/.

20. Pranshu Verma, "The Rise of AI Fake News Is Creating a 'Misinformation Superspreader,'" *Washington Post*, December 17, 2023, https://www.washingtonpost.com/technology/2023/12/17/ai-fake-news-misinformation/.

21. Christopher Doss et al., "Deepfakes and Scientific Knowledge Dissemination," *Scientific Reports* 13 (2023): article 13429, https://doi.org/10.1038/s41598-023-39944-3.

22. Joanne Kenen, "The AI Disinformation Wars," *Politico Nightly*, January 17, 2024, https://www.politico.com/newsletters/politico-nightly/2024/01/17/the-ai-disinformation-wars-00136232.

23. Boudewyns et al., "Awareness of Misinformation in Health-Related Advertising," 38.

24. Center for Countering Digital Hate, *Pandemic Profiteers: The Business of Anti-Vaxx* (Center for Countering Digital Hate, June 1, 2021), 4–6, https://counterhate.com/wp-content/uploads/2022/05/210601-Pandemic-Profiteers-Report.pdf.

25. Center for Countering Digital Hate, *Pandemic Profiteers*, 5.

26. Cass R. Sunstein and Adrian Vermeule, "Conspiracy Theories: Causes and Cures," *Journal of Political Philosophy* 17, no. 2 (2009): 202–27, https://doi.org/10.1111/j.1467-9760.2008.00325.x.

27. Joshua A. Tucker et al., "Social Media, Political Polarization, and Political Disinformation: A Review of the Scientific Literature," Social Science Research Network, March 19, 2018, 3, http://dx.doi.org/10.2139/ssrn.3144139; C. W. Anderson, "Propaganda, Misinformation, and Histories of Media Techniques," *Harvard Kennedy School (HKS) Misinformation Review* 2, no. 2 (2021), https://doi.org/10.37016/mr-2020-64.

28. The Virality Project, *Memes, Magnets and Microchips: Narrative Dynamics Around COVID-19 Vaccines* (2022), Stanford Digital Repository, section 4.3, "Foreign Actors," 96–104, https://doi.org/10.25740/mx395xj8490.

29. Sara E. Gorman, *The Anatomy of Deception: Conspiracy Theories, Distrust, and Public Health in America* (Oxford University Press, 2024), 199.

30. Kaylin Dodson et al., "Covid-19 Vaccine Misinformation and Narratives Surrounding Black Communities on Social Media," First Draft, October 13, 2021, https://firstdraftnews.org/long-form-article/covid-19-vaccine-misinformation-black-communities/. First Draft, a pioneering disinformation research project, has closed but the work has continued at the Information Futures Lab at Brown's School of Public Health.

31. Scott Atlas, "Stanford's Censorship: An Interview with Dr. Scott Atlas," interview by Aadi Golchha and Elsa Johnson, *The Stanford Review*, May 8, 2024, https://stanfordreview.org/stanfords-censorship-an-interview-with-dr-scott-atlas/.

32. Kate Chesley, "Faculty Senate Condemns COVID-19 Actions of Hoover's Scott Atlas," *Stanford Report*, November 20, 2020, https://news.stanford.edu/2020/11/20/faculty-senate-condemns-actions-hoover-fellow-scott-atlas/.

33. Noah Weiland et al., "A New Coronavirus Adviser Roils the White House with Unorthodox Ideas," *New York Times*, September 2, 2020, https://www.nytimes.com/2020/09/02/us/politics/trump-scott-atlas-coronavirus.html.

34. Sandra L. Decker and Samuel H. Zuvekas, "Primary Care Spending in the US Population," *JAMA Internal Medicine* 183, no. 8 (2023): 880–81, https://doi.org/10.1001/jamainternmed.2023.1551.

35. Grace Sparks et al., "KFF COVID-19 Vaccine Monitor: April 2022," KFF, May 4, 2022, https://www.kff.org/coronavirus-covid-19/poll-finding/kff-covid-19-vaccine-monitor-april-2022/.

36. Annie Sundelson et al., *Infodemic Management Approaches Leading Up to, During, and Following the COVID-19 Pandemic* (Johns Hopkins Center for Health Security, March 2023), 3, https://centerforhealthsecurity.org/sites/default/files/2023-04/230407-nasempaper.pdf.

37. Randy Stein and Caroline Meyersohn, "Readers Are More Suspicious of Journalists Providing Corrections Than Journalists Providing Confirmation," Nieman Lab, August 6, 2024, https://www.niemanlab.org/2024/08/readers-are-more-suspicious-of-journalists-providing-corrections-than-journalists-providing-confirmations/.

38. Glenn Kessler, "Meet the Bottomless Pinocchio, a New Rating for a False Claim Repeated over and over Again," *Washington Post*, December 10, 2018, https://www.washingtonpost.com/politics/2018/12/10/meet-bottomless-pinocchio-new-rating-false-claim-repeated-over-over-again/; Glenn Kessler, "A Bottomless Pinocchio for Biden—and Other Recent Gaffes," *Washington Post*, November 7, 2022, https://www.washingtonpost.com/politics/2022/11/07/bottomless-pinocchio-biden-other-recent-gaffes/.

39. Salvador Rizzo, "Four Pinocchios for Ron Johnson's Campaign of Vaccine Misinformation," *Washington Post*, July 16, 2021, https://www.washingtonpost.com/politics/2021/07/16/four-pinocchios-ron-johnsons-campaign-vaccine-misinformation/.

40. Graph Massara, "Combination COVID and Flu Test Does Not Prove They Are the Same Virus," AP News, December 30, 2022, https://apnews.com/article/fact-check-covid-test-flu-virus-396443166714.

41. Graph Massara, classroom interview, November 28, 2022.

42. Massara, classroom interview.

43. Massara, classroom interview.

44. Robert Farley, "Bogus Meme Targets Trump," FactCheck.org, September 28, 2016, https://www.factcheck.org/2015/11/bogus-meme-targets-trump/.

45. Kate Yandell, "Injection Protects Babies from RSV Hospitalization, Has Not Been Linked to Deaths," FactCheck.org, September 25, 2023, https://www.factcheck.org/2023/08/scicheck-injection-protects-babies-from-rsv-hospitalization-has-not-been-linked-to-deaths/.

46. See for example Jessica McDonald, "RFK Jr. Misleads on Vitamin A, Unsupported Therapies for Measles," FactCheck,org, March 7, 2025, https://www.factcheck.org/2025/03/rfk-jr-misleads-on-vitamin-a-unsupported-therapies-for-measles; and McDonald, "Measles Is Harmful, Contrary to Fismy Social Media

Claims of Long-Term Benefits," FactCheck.org, March 14, 2025, https://www.fact check.org/2025/03/measles-is-harmful-contrary-to-flimsy-social-media-claims-of-long-term-benefits/.

47. Ciara O'Rourke, "Former Secretary of State Hillary Clinton Wasn't Executed, but These Zombie Claims Won't Die," PolitiFact, September 21, 2023, https://www.politifact.com/factchecks/2023/sep/21/facebook-posts/former-secretary-of-state-hillary-clinton-wasnt-ex/.

48. "Fighting the Infodemic: The #CoronaVirusFacts Alliance," Poynter Institute, accessed September 24, 2023, https://www.poynter.org/coronavirusfactsalliance/.

49. "English," Factchequeado, accessed February 10, 2025, https://factchequeado.com/english/.

50. Laura Zommer (cofounder, Factchequeado), in discussion with Joanne Kenen, October 18, 2023.

51. Mark Stencel and Erica Ryan, *From Fact Deserts to Fact Streams: Expanding State and Local Fact-Checking in the U.S.* (Duke Reporters' Lab, March 2023).

52. Mark Stencel et al., "Vast Gaps in Fact-Checking Across the U.S. Allow Politicians to Elude Scrutiny," Duke Reporters' Lab, March 29, 2023, https://reporterslab.org/vast-gaps-in-fact-checking-across-the-u-s-allow-politicians-to-elude-scrutiny/.

53. Joanne Kenen, "How to Wage War on Conspiracy Theories," *Politico Nightly*, September 5, 2023, https://www.politico.com/newsletters/politico-nightly/2023/09/05/how-to-wage-war-on-conspiracy-theories-00114093.

54. Bill Adair, "The Lessons of Squash, Our Groundbreaking Automated Fact-Checking Platform," Duke Reporters' Lab, June 28, 2021, https://reporterslab.org/the-lessons-of-squash-our-groundbreaking-automated-fact-checking-platform/.

55. Emily Breza et al., "Effects of a Large-Scale Social Media Advertising Campaign on Holiday Travel and COVID-19 Infections: A Cluster Randomized Controlled Trial," *Nature Medicine* 27, no. 9 (2021): 1622–28, https://doi.org/10.1038/s41591-021-01487-3.

56. Alex Moehring et al., "Providing Normative Information Increases Intentions to Accept a COVID-19 Vaccine," *Nature Communications* 14, no. 1 (2023), https://doi.org/10.1038/s41467-022-35052-4.

57. Marcella Alsan et al., "Comparison of Knowledge and Information-Seeking Behavior After General COVID-19 Public Health Messages and Messages Tailored for Black and Latinx Communities: A Randomized Controlled Trial," *Annals of Internal Medicine* 174, no. 4 (2021): 484–92, https://doi.org/10.7326/m20-6141.

58. Adam J. Berinsky, *Political Rumors: Why We Accept Misinformation and How to Fight It* (Princeton University Press, 2023), 82.

59. Fabiana Zollo et al., "Debunking in a World of Tribes," *PLoS ONE* 12, no. 7 (2017): e0181821, https://doi.org/10.1371/journal.pone.0181821.

60. Wei-Yang Chou et al., "The COVID-19 Misinfodemic: Moving Beyond Fact-Checking," *Health Education and Behavior* 48, no. 1 (2020): 10, https://doi.org/10.1177/1090198120980675.

61. DROG et al., "Bad News—Play the Fake News Game!," Bad News, February 19, 2018, https://www.getbadnews.com/en/.

62. Bob Ward, "Foolproof by Sander van Der Linden Review—How to Defuse Fake News," *Guardian*, February 12, 2023, https://www.theguardian.com/books/2023/feb/12/foolproof-by-sander-van-der-linden-review-how-to-defuse-fake-news; Beth Goldberg, "Inoculation Theory: A Beginners Guide," Inoculation Science, 2021, https://inoculation.science/inoculation-theory-a-beginners-guide/.

63. Polarization and Extremism Research and Innovation Lab (PERIL), home page, American University, School of Public Affairs, accessed February 10, 2025, https://www.american.edu/spa/peril/.

64. "Training," First Draft, accessed January 29, 2024, https://firstdraftnews.org/training/.

65. Trisha Harjani et al., *A Practical Guide to Prebunking Misinformation* (University of Cambridge, BBC Media Action, and Jigsaw, 2022), 8–9, https://interventions.withgoogle.com/static/pdf/A_Practical_Guide_to_Prebunking_Misinformation.pdf.

66. Goldberg, "Inoculation Theory."

67. Zommer, in discussion with Kenen.

68. The Virality Project, *Memes, Magnets and Microchips: Narrative Dynamics Around COVID-19 Vaccines* (2022), Stanford Digital Repository, section 1, "Introduction," 10–14, and section 3, "Narratives," 42–73, https://doi.org/10.25740/mx395xj8490.

69. This particular video, which the authors have viewed, seems to have been taken down or is no longer easiy found in a search. But there were quite a few similar videos about parasites, hydras and creatures with tentacles. Reuters is one of several organization that fact-checked such claims. "Fact Check: COVID-19 Vaccines Do Not Contain Live Immortal Creatures, Experts Say," Reuters, October 26, 2021, https://www.reuters.com/article/fact-check/covid-19-vaccines-do-not-contain-live-immortal-creatures-experts-say-idUSL1N2RM2F3/.

70. Dave Chokshi (health commissioner, New York City Department of Health and Mental Hygiene), in discussion with Joanne Kenen, March 11, 2022.

71. Chokshi, in discussion with Kenen.

72. Matthew Kreuter (Kahn Family Professor of Public Health, Brown School of Public Health, Washington University, St. Louis), in discussion with Joanne Kenen, October 18, 2023.

73. Reed Tuckson (chair and cofounder, Black Coalition Against Covid), in discussion with Joanne Kenen, October 27, 2023.

74. Katy Evans (senior program officer, de Beaumont Foundation), in discussion with Joanne Kenen, November 8, 2023.

75. Drew Altman, "KFF's New Health Misinformation and Trust Initiative," KFF, June 13, 2024, https://www.kff.org/kffs-new-health-misinformation-and-trust-initiative/.

76. Ezra Klein, "Is the Government Going to Euthanize Your Grandmother? An Interview with Sen. Johnny Isakson," *Washington Post*, August 10, 2009, archived March 28, 2011, https://web.archive.org/web/20110328191405/http://voices.washingtonpost.com/ezra-klein/2009/08/is_the_government_going_to_eut.html. Even though Republicans uniformly voted against the Affordable Care Act, some legislative measures they had authored or coauthored that had bipartisan support were incorporated into the massive health law.

77. Berinsky, *Political Rumors*, 91–95.

78. Lunna Lopes et al., "KFF Health Misinformation Tracking Poll Pilot," KFF, August 22, 2023, https://www.kff.org/coronavirus-covid-19/poll-finding/kff-health-misinformation-tracking-poll-pilot/.

79. "Authoritative Health Information," YouTube, accessed January 21, 2024, https://www.youtube.com/howyoutubeworks/product-features/health-information/#raising-authoritative-health-sources.

80. Raynard S. Kington et al., "Identifying Credible Sources of Health Information in Social Media: Principles and Attributes," *NAM Perspectives*, July 16, 2021, https://doi.org/10.31478/202107a.

81. ABIM Foundation, *2022 ABIM Foundation Forum Summary Paper: Fact or Fiction Strategies for the Misinformation Age* (ABIM Foundation, 2022), 7, https://abimfoundation.org/wp-content/uploads/2022/09/Summary_Paper_2022.pdf.

82. Helen Burstin et al., "Identifying Credible Sources of Health Information in Social Media: Phase 2—Considerations for Non-Accredited Nonprofit Organizations, For-Profit Entities, and Individual Sources," *NAM Perspectives*, May 23, 2023, https://doi.org/10.31478/202305b.

83. "Biden's 'Ministry of Truth' on Pause," Office of Congresswoman Cathy McMorris Rodgers, May 20, 2022, https://mcmorris.house.gov/posts/bidens-ministry-of-truth-on-pause.

84. Shannon Bond, "She Joined DHS to Fight Disinformation. She Says She Was Halted by . . . Disinformation," NPR, May 21, 2022, https://www.npr.org/2022/05/21/1100438703/dhs-disinformation-board-nina-jankowicz.

85. Black Coalition Against COVID, home page, accessed April 21, 2024, https://blackcoalitionagainstcovid.org.

86. Made to Save, home page, accessed April 21, 2024, https://madetosave.org.

87. Nitish Pahwa, "What I Saw in Elon Musk's Truth Army," *Slate*, July 10, 2023, https://slate.com/technology/2023/07/twitter-community-notes-elon-musk-fact-checking.html.

88. Thomas Germain, "Twitter Users Vote Down a Note Correcting Elon's Bogus Vaccine Tweets," Gizmodo, July 26, 2023, https://gizmodo.com/twitter-x-elon-musk-vaccine-bronny-james-fact-check-1850678981; Matias Grez, "LeBron James

Says Son Bronny Is 'Doing Extremely Well' After Cardiac Arrest and Aims to Play This Season," CNN, October 3, 2023, https://www.cnn.com/2023/10/03/sport/lebron-james-son-bronny-doing-extremely-well-after-cardiac-arrest-and-aims-to-play-this-season/index.html.

89. Brandy Zadrozny, host, *Truthers: Tiffany Dover Is Dead*, podcast, season 1, episode 3, "Who Does That?," NBC News, April 25, 2022, https://podcasts.apple.com/us/podcast/who-does-that/id1618512442?i=1000558584581.

90. Zadrozny, "Who Does That?"

Chapter 4. The Innovators

1. Alissa Zhu, classroom interview, November 7, 2022.
2. Andrea K. McDaniels, classroom interview, April 6, 2022.
3. McDaniels, classroom interview.
4. Katie Robertson, "Is Baltimore Big Enough for the Two of Them?," *New York Times*, July 2, 2022, https://www.nytimes.com/2022/07/01/business/media/baltimore-banner-the-sun.html; Rick Edmonds, "A Philanthropist Pivots: How Stewart Bainum Jr. Came to Pledge $50 Million to Launch the Baltimore Banner," Poynter, February 10, 2022, https://www.poynter.org/business-work/2022/philanthropist-stewart-bainum-jr-launch-baltimore-banner/.
5. McDaniels, classroom interview.
6. McDaniels, classroom interview.
7. Alissa Zhu et al., "Almost 6,000 Dead in 6 Years: How Baltimore Became the U.S. Overdose Capital," *New York Times*, May 23, 2024. This was part of a multipart series.
8. "Index Snapshot Report 2023: The State of Nonprofit News," Institute for Nonprofit News, May 23, 2023, https://inn.org/research/inn-index/inn-index-2023/.
9. Charles Ornstein, classroom interview, May 4, 2022.
10. Ornstein, classroom interview.
11. Ornstein, classroom interview.
12. Caroline Chen (reporter, ProPublica), in email correspondence with Joanne Kenen, January 3, 2024. See Caroline Chen, "'It's Very Unethical': Audio Shows Hospital Kept Vegetative Patient on Life Support to Boost Survival Rates," ProPublica, October 3, 2019, https://www.propublica.org/article/audio-shows-hospital-kept-vegetative-patient-on-life-support-to-boost-survival-rates. Chen later left journalism, at least for a while, for family reasons.
13. Drew Altman (president and CEO, KFF), in discussion with Joanne Kenen, August 22, 2023.
14. Coauthor Joanne Kenen was a Kaiser media fellow in 2006–7, has been a regular panelist on KFF's *What the Health* blog since its inception, and has been a contributor to KFF Health News.
15. Altman, in discussion with Kenen.
16. Jane Spencer et al., "12 Months of Trauma: More Than 3,600 US Health Workers Died in Covid's First Year," KFF Health News, April 8, 2021, https://

kffhealthnews.org/news/article/us-health-workers-deaths-covid-lost-on-the-frontline/; *Guardian* and Kaiser Health News, "Lost on the Frontline," *Guardian*, April 8, 2021, https://www.theguardian.com/us-news/series/lost-on-the-frontline; Noam Levey et al., "Diagnosis: Debt," KFF Health News, accessed December 30, 2023, https://kffhealthnews.org/diagnosis-debt/.

17. "Dying Broke," *New York Times*, accessed December 30, 2023, https://www.nytimes.com/series/dying-broke; Jordan Rau et al., "Dying Broke," KFF Health News, accessed December 30, 2023, https://kffhealthnews.org/dying-broke/.

18. David Rousseau, prerecorded classroom lecture, May 1, 2022.

19. Rousseau, prerecorded classroom lecture.

20. Altman, in discussion with Kenen.

21. Eyre, for both personal and professional reasons, didn't stay with Mountain Spotlight; he disclosed his early-onset Parkinson's disease as he was writing *Death in Mud Lick*, a book recounting the role of the drug distributors in the opioid epidemic, and the war waged on the *Gazette-Mail* as it tried to expose it. He's been working on projects related to the book and writing an oral history of the opioid epidemic for the state's humanities council. More recently, he began contributing to West Virginia Watch, a second nonprofit created by *Gazette-Mail* alumni, which is part of the States Newsroom described later. Both of the nonprofits are devoting a fair amount of their time to covering health in a state with an opioid crisis and a high burden of chronic disease.

22. The Marshall Project, *Changing the Narrative on Criminal Justice Annual Report 2015* (The Marshall Project, 2015), https://s3.amazonaws.com/tmp-uploads-2/reports/2015-Annual-Report.pdf; The Marshall Project, *Financial Statements and Supplementary Information: December 31, 2015 and 2014* (The Marshall Project, 2015), https://tmp-uploads-2.s3.amazonaws.com/financials/2015-Financial-Statements.pdf; Rick Edmonds, "Mission Accomplished at the Marshall Project? Why Founder Neil Barsky Is Moving On After 7 Years," Poynter, December 7, 2021, https://www.poynter.org/business-work/2021/mission-accomplished-at-the-marshall-project-why-founder-neil-barsky-is-moving-on-after-7-years/.

23. Beth Schwartzapfel, classroom interview, May 4, 2022.

24. Schwartzapfel, classroom interview.

25. Katie Park et al., "A Half-Million People Got COVID-19 in Prison. Are Officials Ready for the Next Pandemic?," The Marshall Project, June 30, 2021, https://www.themarshallproject.org/2021/06/30/a-half-million-people-got-covid-19-in-prison-are-officials-ready-for-the-next-pandemic.

26. The Trace, accessed March 12, 2025, https://www.thetrace.org/about-the-trace/.

27. J. Brian Charles, classroom interview, May 4, 2022.

28. J. Brian Charles, "The Human Toll of Keeping Baltimore Safe," The Trace, March 3, 2022, https://www.thetrace.org/2022/03/baltimore-safe-streets-shootings-gun-violence-mayor-scott/.

29. Fairriona Magee, "Gun Violence Isn't an Isolated Crisis. Its Solutions Aren't Isolated, Either," interview by Sunny Sone, The Trace, June 16, 2023, https://www.thetrace.org/newsletter/gun-violence-american-crisis-solutions/.

30. Fairriona Magee, classroom interview, December 12, 2022.

31. Sam Fromartz, classroom interviews, May 4 and December 12, 2022.

32. Fromartz, classroom interviews, May 4 and December 12, 2022.

33. Fromartz, classroom interviews, May 4 and December 12, 2022.

34. Fromartz, classroom interviews, May 4 and December 12, 2022.

35. Fromartz, classroom interview, May 4, 2022.

36. Documenters, home page, City Bureau, accessed January 1, 2024, https://www.documenters.org/.

37. Chris Fitzsimon (director and publisher, States Newsroom), in discussion with Joanne Kenen, September 7, 2023.

38. Jessica Mahone and Philip Napoli, "Hundreds of Hyperpartisan Sites Are Masquerading as Local News. This Map Shows If There's One Near You," Nieman Lab, July 13, 2020, https://www.niemanlab.org/2020/07/hundreds-of-hyperpartisan-sites-are-masquerading-as-local-news-this-map-shows-if-theres-one-near-you/. See the note appended to the bottom of this article about the funding controversy.

39. "Pew's Stateline to Join States Newsroom," States Newsroom, March 8, 2023, https://statesnewsroom.com/press-releases/pews-stateline-to-join-states-newsroom/.

40. Fitzsimon, in discussion with Kenen.

41. Fitzsimon, in discussion with Kenen.

42. Jeanne Pinder (founder and CEO, ClearHealthCosts), in discussion with Joanne Kenen, September 26, 2023.

43. Pinder, in discussion with Kenen.

44. Pinder, in discussion with Kenen.

45. Lee Zurik and Tom Wright, "Zurik: 'Cracking the Code' of Medical Procedure Pricing," FOX8 Live, April 6, 2017, https://www.fox8live.com/story/35080698/zurik-cracking-the-code-of-medical-procedure-pricing/.

46. Peter S. Hussey et al., "The Association Between Health Care Quality and Cost: A Systematic Review," *Annals of Internal Medicine* 158, no. 1 (2013): 27–34, https://doi.org/10.7326/0003-4819-158-1-201301010-00006.

47. Pinder, in discussion with Kenen.

48. "Philanthropy's Growing Role in American Journalism: A New Study Reveals Increased Funding and Ethical Considerations," Media Impact Funders, August 23, 2023, https://mediaimpactfunders.org/philanthropys-growing-role-in-american-journalism-a-new-study-reveals-increased-funding-and-ethical-considerations/.

49. "Philanthropy's Growing Role in American Journalism."

50. Zhu, classroom interview.

Chapter 5. By and For

1. Dianna Hunt, classroom interview, April 27, 2022.

2. Hunt, classroom interview; Dianna Hunt (senior editor, ICT), in discussion with Joanne Kenen, September 12, 2023.

3. Penelope Muse Abernathy et al., *News Deserts and Ghost Newspapers: Will Local News Survive?* (Center for Innovation and Sustainability in Local Media, June 2020), 57–59, https://www.usnewsdeserts.com/wp-content/uploads/2020/06/2020_News_Deserts_and_Ghost_Newspapers.pdf.

4. Lautaro Grinspan, "How Spanish-Language Radio Helped Radicalize a Generation of Miami Abuelos," *HuffPost*, October 21, 2021, https://www.huffpost.com/entry/miami-spanish-language-radio-misinformation_n_616dbd3ee4b005b245c0b57e; Gabriel R. Sanchez and Keesha Middlemass, "Misinformation Is Eroding the Public's Confidence in Democracy," Brookings, July 26, 2022, https://www.brookings.edu/articles/misinformation-is-eroding-the-publics-confidence-in-democracy/; Whitney Tesi, "When Disinformation Becomes 'Racialized,'" ABC News, February 5, 2022, https://abcnews.go.com/Technology/disinformation-racialized/story?id=82400863; Kaylin Dodson et al., "Covid-19 Vaccine Misinformation and Narratives Surrounding Black Communities on Social Media," First Draft, October 13, 2021, https://firstdraftnews.org/long-form-article/covid-19-vaccine-misinformation-black-communities/; Jaime Longoria et al., "A Limiting Lens: How Vaccine Misinformation Has Influenced Hispanic Conversations Online," First Draft, December 8, 2021, https://firstdraftnews.org/long-form-article/covid19-vaccine-misinformation-hispanic-latinx-social-media/.

5. Gene Roberts and Hank Klibanoff, *The Race Beat: The Press, the Civil Rights Struggle, and the Awakening of a Nation* (Vintage, 2006).

6. Quoted in PEN America, *Losing the News: The Decimation of Local Journalism and the Search for Solutions* (PEN America, November 20, 2019), 34, https://pen.org/wp-content/uploads/2024/07/2019_Losing-the-News-The-Decimation-of-Local-Journalism-and-the-Search-for-Solutions-Report.pdf.

7. "Index Report on Diversity, Equity, and Inclusion in the Nonprofit News Sector," Institute for Nonprofit News, October 24, 2023, https://inn.org/research/inn-index/dei-report-on-diversity-equity-and-inclusion-in-the-nonprofit-news-sector/race-ethnicity/.

8. *Freedom's Journal*, March 16, 1827.

9. Larry Muhammad, "The Black Press: Past and Present," *Nieman Reports*, September 15, 2003, https://niemanreports.org/the-black-press-past-and-present/.

10. PEN America, *Losing the News*, 33.

11. PEN America, *Losing the News*, 34.

12. Cheryl Thompson-Morton, "Introduction," Why Black Media Matters Now, accessed March 24, 2023, https://blackmediareport.journalism.cuny.edu/.

13. Thompson-Morton, "Introduction."

14. Sara Guaglione, "Despite DEI Promises, Media Companies Are Still Mostly Hiring White People," *Digiday*, April 18, 2023, https://digiday.com/media/despite-dei-promises-media-companies-are-still-mostly-hiring-white-people/.

15. Elahe Izadi, "'A Community Deserves Options': Why These Black Journalists Launched Their Own Publication," *Washington Post*, January 31, 2022, https://www.washingtonpost.com/media/2022/01/31/capital-b-black-media/.

16. "Knight Foundation Announces Investment in Publishers of Color to Foster Their Digital Transformation, Sustainability," Knight Foundation, February 21, 2022, https://knightfoundation.org/press/releases/knight-foundation-announces-investment-in-publishers-of-color-to-foster-their-digital-transformation-sustainability/.

17. Sarah Scire, "Capital B, Written for and by Black People, Launches as a Nonprofit Newsroom," Nieman Lab, February 1, 2022, https://www.niemanlab.org/2022/02/capital-b-written-for-and-by-black-people-launches-as-a-nonprofit-newsroom/.

18. Lauren Williams and Akoto Ofori-Atta, "Why It's the Right Time for a Capital B," Capital B, January 31, 2022, https://capitalbnews.org/welcome-introduction-cofounders/.

19. Margo Snipe, "All About Margo Snipe," Capital B, February 2, 2022, https://capitalbnews.org/margo-snipe-staff-intro/.

20. Margo Snipe, "Misinformation Is on the Rise. Here's What You Need to Know About Birth Control," Capital B, March 25, 2024, https://capitalbnews.org/birth-control-misinformation/.

21. Elizabeth Arias et al., "Mortality Profile of the Non-Hispanic American Indian or Alaska Native Population, 2019," *National Vital Statistics Reports* 70, no. 12 (2021): 2, https://doi.org/10.15620/cdc:110370.

22. Jessica L. Garcia, "Historical Trauma and American Indian / Alaska Native Youth Mental Health Development and Delinquency," *New Directions for Child and Adolescent Development* 2020, no. 169 (2020): 41–58, https://doi.org/10.1002/cad.20332.

23. "American Indian / Alaska Native Health," Office of Minority Health, accessed June 5, 2023, https://minorityhealth.hhs.gov/american-indianalaska-native-health; Adali Martinez et al., "Structural Racism and Its Pathways to Asthma and Atopic Dermatitis," *Journal of Allergy and Clinical Immunology* 148, no. 5 (2021): 1112–20, https://doi.org/10.1016/j.jaci.2021.09.020.

24. Jamie E. Ehrenpreis and Eli D. Ehrenpreis, "A Historical Perspective of Healthcare Disparity and Infectious Disease in the Native American Population," *American Journal of the Medical Sciences* 363, no. 4 (2022): 288–94, https://doi.org/10.1016/j.amjms.2022.01.005.

25. Amanda Hinnant et al., "How Journalists Characterize Health Inequalities and Redefine Solutions for Native American Audiences," *Health Communication* 34, no. 4 (2019): 383–91, https://doi.org/10.1080/10410236.2017.1405482.

26. Gemma DiCarlo, "New Indian Health Service Funding Provides Stability, but Long-Standing Issues Remain," OPB, January 23, 2023, https://www.opb.org

/article/2023/01/20/new-indian-health-service-funding-provides-stability-but-long-standing-issues-remain/; Ehrenpreis and Ehrenpreis, "Historical Perspective."

27. Hunt, classroom interview.

28. Jenni Monet, "The Crisis in Covering Indian Country," *Columbia Journalism Review*, March 29, 2019, https://www.cjr.org/opinion/indigenous-journalism-erasure.php.

29. Monet, "Crisis in Covering Indian Country."

30. Hunt, classroom interview.

31. "Federally Recognized Indian Tribes and Resources for Native Americans," USA.gov, accessed June 5, 2023, https://www.usa.gov/tribes.

32. Hunt, classroom interview.

33. Hunt, classroom interview.

34. Steve Dubb, "Indian Country Today's Future Is Bright After Near-Death Experience," *Nonprofit Quarterly*, June 16, 2021, https://nonprofitquarterly.org/indian-country-todays-future-is-bright-after-near-death-experience/.

35. "Rural News Network to Launch Projects Centering Indigenous Communities and Water Access," Institute for Nonprofit News, November 17, 2021, https://inn.org/news/rural-news-network-to-launch-projects-centering-indigenous-communities-and-water-access/.

36. "National Health Care Group Seeds INN's Next Rural Health Collaboration," Institute for Nonprofit News, March 24, 2023, https://inn.org/news/national-health-care-group-seeds-inns-next-rural-health-collaboration/.

37. Hunt, classroom interview.

38. "Welcome to the 19th*," The 19th, accessed June 8, 2023, https://19thnews.org/about/.

39. Abby Johnston, classroom interview, April 27, 2022.

40. Katie Robertson, "After Roe v. Wade Reversal, Readers Flock to Publications Aimed at Women," *New York Times*, August 14, 2022, https://www.nytimes.com/2022/08/14/business/media/abortion-womens-media.html.

41. Johnston, classroom interview.

42. Johnston, classroom interview.

43. Johnston, classroom interview.

44. Shefali Luthra, classroom interview, December 5, 2022.

45. Luthra, classroom interview.

46. Luthra, classroom interview.

47. Luthra, classroom interview.

48. Luthra, classroom interview.

49. Luthra, classroom interview.

50. Luthra, classroom interview.

51. Wayne Shoaf, "Spanish-Language Newspapers from El MisisipÃ to El Clamor PÃºblico," USC Libraries, March 16, 2009, https://libraries.usc.edu/article/spanish-language-newspapers-el-misisip%C3%A3%C2%AD-el-clamor-p%C3%A3%C2%BAblico.

52. "The Industry at a Glance," in *The State of the Latino News Media* (City University of New York Craig Newmark Graduate School of Journalism, June 2019), https://thelatinomediareport.journalism.cuny.edu/the-industry-at-a-glance/.

53. "Industry at a Glance."

54. *Tostada Magazine*, home page, accessed June 9, 2023, https://tostadamagazine.com/o; PEN America, *Losing the News*, 42.

55. Serena Maria Daniels, email to authors, June 9, 2023.

56. Luz Gray, classroom interviews, April 27 and December 5, 2022.

57. Gray, classroom interviews.

58. "Industry at a Glance."

59. Gray, classroom interviews.

60. Gray, classroom interviews.

61. Gray, classroom interviews.

62. Gray, classroom interviews.

63. Gray, classroom interviews.

64. Gray, classroom interviews.

65. Gray, classroom interviews.

66. Gray, classroom interviews.

67. Gray, classroom interviews.

68. Luthra, classroom interview.

69. Hunt, classroom interview.

Chapter 6. The Playbook

1. Renée DiResta, *Invisible Rulers: The People Who Turn Lies into Reality* (Public Affairs, 2024), 3–11.

2. See, e.g., "Changing the COVID Conversation," de Beaumont Foundation, accessed February 11, 2025, https://debeaumont.org/changing-the-covid-conversation/; Public Good Projects, home page, accessed February 11, 2025, https://www.publicgoodprojects.org/; and "Messaging Research: Effective Public Health Communication Strategies for Divisive Political Climate," Big Cities Health Coalition, accessed February 11, 2025, https://www.bigcitieshealth.org/public-health-changing-narrative/.

3. This Is Our Shot, home page, accessed February 11, 2025, https://thisisourshot.info/.

4. Irving Washington and Hagere Yilma, "Raw Milk Myths, Vaccine Falsehoods, and Reproductive Health Narratives," KFF *Health Misinformation Monitor* 1 (June 13, 2024), https://www.kff.org/health-misinformation-monitor/volume-01/.

5. Lydia Saad, "Historically Low Faith in U.S. Institutions Continues," Gallup, July 6, 2023, https://news.gallup.com/poll/508169/historically-low-faith-institutions-continues.aspx; Megan Brenan, "Americans' Confidence in Higher Education Down Sharply," Gallup, July 11, 2023, https://news.gallup.com/poll/508352/americans-confidence-higher-education-down-sharply.aspx.

6. Shima Hamidi and Reid Ewing, *A National Investigation on the Impacts of Lane Width on Traffic Safety: Narrowing Travel Lanes as an Opportunity to Promote Biking and Pedestrian Facilities Within the Existing Roadway Infrastructure* (Bloomberg American Health Initiative, November 2023), https://narrowlanes.americanhealth.jhu.edu/report/JHU-2023-Narrowing-Travel-Lanes-Report.pdf.

7. Rupali Limaye et al., "How Can I Talk to My Friends and Family About Getting Vaccinated for COVID-19?," Johns Hopkins Bloomberg School of Public Health, May 6, 2021, https://publichealth.jhu.edu/2021/how-can-i-talk-to-my-friends-and-family-about-getting-vaccinated-for-covid-19; Johns Hopkins Bloomberg School of Public Health (@johnshopkinssph), "Need Some Helpful Tips on How to Talk to Your Friends and Family About Getting the COVID-19 Vaccine? We've Got You Covered!," Instagram, May 17, 2021, https://www.instagram.com/p/CO-vLoALQmY/?img_index=1; Johns Hopkins Bloomberg School of Public Health (@johnshopkinssph), "¿Necesita algunos consejos útiles sobre cómo hablar con sus amigos y familiares sobre la vacuna COVID-19? Te tenemos cubierto!," Instagram, May 19, 2021, https://www.instagram.com/p/CPD3ouNLwKg/?img_index=1; Johns Hopkins Bloomberg School of Public Health (@johnshopkinssph), "Sometimes Talking to Friends and Family About Vaccines Can Be Difficult, So We've Got You Covered. Here Are Some Helpful Tips on How to Talk to Rhem About Getting Vaccinated," Instagram, May 21, 2021, https://www.instagram.com/p/CPI_lHhLHAU/?img_index=1; Johns Hopkins Bloomberg School of Public Health (@johnshopkinssph), "A veces, puede ser difícil hablar con amigos y familiares sobre las vacunas, así que te tenemos cubierto. Aquí están algunos consejos útiles sobre cómo hablar con ellos sobre la vacunación," Instagram, May 24, 2021, https://www.instagram.com/p/CPQt7taLzjz/?img_index=1.

8. "Safe and Secure Gun Storage," Center for Gun Violence Solutions, Johns Hopkins Bloomberg School of Public Health, accessed January 29, 2024, https://publichealth.jhu.edu/departments/health-policy-and-management/research-and-practice/center-for-gun-violence-solutions/solutions/safe-and-secure-gun-storage.

9. Cassandra K. Crifasi et al., "Storage Practices of US Gun Owners in 2016," *American Journal of Public Health* 108, no. 4 (2018): 532–37, https://doi.org/10.2105/ajph.2017.304262.

10. Aliza Rosen, "Locked and UN-Loaded: The Importance of Safe and Secure Firearm Storage," Johns Hopkins Bloomberg School of Public Health, May 25, 2023, https://publichealth.jhu.edu/2023/how-safe-and-secure-gun-storage-reduces-injury-saves-lives; Aliza Rosen, "Yes, You Should Ask If Someone Has Guns in the Home. Here's How," Johns Hopkins Bloomberg School of Public Health, May 30, 2023, https://publichealth.jhu.edu/2023/why-and-how-you-should-ask-other-parents-if-they-own-guns.

11. Johns Hopkins Bloomberg School of Public Health (@johnshopkinssph), "Planning a Playdate? Let's Normalize Asking About Firearm Storage in the Same Judgment-Free Way We Do Other Safety Issues, like Allergens, Pets, or Whether

the Backyard Is Fenced. Asking About Guns in the Home Can Feel Awkward, but It Doesn't have to Be," Instagram, May 30, 2023, https://www.instagram.com/p/Cs31XtcMpDL/?img_index=5.

12. Heather Hollingsworth, "Doctors Grow Frustrated over COVID-19 Denial, Misinformation," AP News, October 4, 2021, https://apnews.com/article/coronavirus-pandemic-misinformation-health-433991ea434e12ccfdf97b5db415310d.

13. John Robert Bautista et al., "US Physicians' and Nurses' Motivations, Barriers, and Recommendations for Correcting Health Misinformation on Social Media: Qualitative Interview Study," *JMIR Public Health and Surveillance* 7, no. 9 (2021): e27715, https://doi.org/10.2196/27715.

14. Mehdi Mourali and Carly Drake, "The Challenge of Debunking Health Misinformation in Dynamic Social Media Conversations: Online Randomized Study of Public Masking During COVID-19," *Journal of Medical Internet Research* 24, no. 3 (2022): e34831, https://doi.org/10.2196/34831.

15. Bautista et al., "US Physicians' and Nurses' Motivations."

16. Daniel A. Salmon et al., "*LetsTalkShots*: Personalized Vaccine Risk Communication," *Frontiers in Public Health* 11 (June 30, 2023), https://doi.org/10.3389/fpubh.2023.1195751, erratum in *Frontiers in Public Health* 11 (October 30, 2023), https://doi.org/10.3389/fpubh.2023.1311055.

17. Matthew Z. Dudley et al., "MomsTalkShots, Tailored Educational App, Improves Vaccine Attitudes: A Randomized Controlled Trial," *BMC Public Health* 22, no. 1 (2022): article 2134, https://doi.org/10.1186/s12889-022-14498-7; Saad B. Omer et al., "Multi-Tiered Intervention to Increase Maternal Immunization Coverage: A Randomized, Controlled Trial," *Vaccine* 40, no. 34 (2022): 4955–63, https://doi.org/10.1016/j.vaccine.2022.06.055.

18. Shikha Jain et al., "Empowering Health Care Workers on Social Media to Bolster Trust in Science and Vaccination During the Pandemic: Making IMPACT Using a Place-Based Approach," *Journal of Medical Internet Research* 24, no. 10 (2022): e38949, https://doi.org/10.2196/38949.

19. Catherine Buni, "Meet the States Using Public Funding to Support Local Journalism," Nieman Reports, February 8, 2023, https://niemanreports.org/articles/state-public-funding-local-news/.

20. Lindsey Graham and Elizabeth Warren, "Lindsey Graham and Elizabeth Warren: We Must Regulate Big Tech," *New York Times*, July 27, 2023, https://www.nytimes.com/2023/07/27/opinion/lindsey-graham-elizabeth-warren-big-tech-regulation.html.

Chapter 7. Protecting Yourself—and Others

1. PolitiFact, home page, Poynter Institute, accessed January 18, 2024, https://www.politifact.com/; FactCheck.org, home page, Annenberg Public Policy Center, accessed January 18, 2024, https://www.factcheck.org/.

2. Factchequeado, home page, accessed January 18, 2024, https://www.factchequeado.com/.

3. "International Fact-Checking Network," Poynter Institute, accessed January 18, 2024, https://www.poynter.org/ifcn/.

4. "International Fact-Checking Network"; Glenn Kessler, "Fact Checker: The Truth Behind the Rhetoric," *Washington Post*, accessed January 18, 2024, https://www.washingtonpost.com/politics/fact-checker/.

5. Elizabeth Svoboda, "Vaccinating People Against Fake News," Nieman Lab, September 1, 2022, https://www.niemanlab.org/2022/09/vaccinating-people-against-fake-news/.

6. "News Literacy Tips, Tools and Quizzes," News Literacy Project, accessed January 18, 2024, https://newslit.org/tips-tools/.

7. Alex Mahadevan et al., "MediaWise: Digital Media Literacy for All," Poynter Institute, accessed January 18, 2024, https://www.poynter.org/mediawise/.

8. Trusting News, home page, accessed January 18, 2024, https://trustingnews.org/.

9. NewsGuard, home page, accessed January 18, 2024, https://www.newsguardtech.com/.

10. SciLine, home page, American Association for the Advancement of Science, accessed January 18, 2024, https://www.sciline.org/.

11. ScienceUpFirst, home page, Canadian Association of Science Centres, accessed January 18, 2024, https://www.scienceupfirst.com/.

12. Coalition for Trust in Health and Science, home page, accessed January 18, 2024, https://trustinhealthandscience.org/.

13. "Diseases and Conditions," Mayo Clinic, accessed January 18, 2024, https://www.mayoclinic.org/diseases-conditions.

14. "Health," Johns Hopkins Medicine, accessed January 18, 2024, https://www.hopkinsmedicine.org/health.

15. Molly Beestrum, "Evaluating Sources: C.R.A.P. Test," Houston Community College Libraries, accessed January 18, 2024, https://library.hccs.edu/evaluatingsources/test. One example at the Houston Community College Libraries has both text and slides to explain the system. Other libraries present it slighty differently. See for instance the Colorado Community College System version, CCCOnline, CRAP Test, www.ccconline.org/wp-content/uploads/2016/04/CRAP-Test.pdf.

16. Mike Caulfield, "Evaluating Resources and Misinformation: The SIFT Method," University of Chicago Library, accessed January 18, 2024, https://guides.lib.uchicago.edu/c.php?g=1241077&p=9082322.

INDEX

AAR (Armed American Radio) Daily Defense Hour, 20
abcnews.com.co (fake news site), 25
abortion access, 30–31, 69, 112, 123, 127–28
academic institutions, playbook for, 146–50
accountability, 13–14, 33–35, 38, 54, 78–79, 112, 125
Adams, Jerome, 32, 53
addiction. *See* drug overdose; opioids
Affordable Care Act (ACA, 2010): "death panels," debunking of, 90–91; enrollment glitches and fixes, 58–59; exaggeration of flaws by opponents to, 27–28; expansion of health insurance options, 2; KFF coverage of, 103–4; national news coverage of, 54, 56; Nevada and, 135; polls on, 51–52; reporting challenges of, 12, 22, 28, 41–43; Republicans and, 28, 42, 90–91, 182n76
Air America, 20
Alabama Power, 25
Alabama Reflector, 112
Alden Global Capital, 15–17, 96–97
Alonso-Zaldivar, Ricardo, 7, 41–44, 55, 66
Altman, Drew, 101–2, 104
American Academy of Pediatrics, 92
American Association for the Advancement of Science, 39; SciLine (online resource), 159
American Society of News Editors, 124
American University, Polarization and Extremism Research and Innovation Lab, 87
America's Frontline Doctors, 32
Annenberg Public Policy Center, 3, 81, 157

anti-vaxxers, 68–69, 73–74, 76–77
Apopka Times, 24
Arizona State University, Cronkite School of Journalism and Mass Communication, 126
artificial intelligence (AI), 5, 29, 72, 84, 155, 159
Associated Press, 7, 31, 41–43, 66, 157; fact-checking team, 80, 158; ICT and, 123, 126, 136; Marshall Project partnership, 107
Atlas, Scott, 75
autism, 3, 31, 36, 88
avoiding reporters, as bad strategy, 142–43, 154
Axios, 63

Bad News (online game), 86, 158
Bainum, Stewart, Jr., 97–98
Ballmer Group, 36
Baltimore, 15–19, 98, 107–8, 141
Baltimore Afro-American (newspaper), 121
Baltimore Banner, 7, 16, 98–99, 115–16
Baltimore City Health Department, 145
Baltimore Sun, 15–17, 21, 96–98, 102
Barsky, Neil, 105
Bartelme, Tony, 37–40
Beestrum, Molly, 161
Berinsky, Adam, 51, 85
Besser, Richard, 52–53, 58
Bezos, Jeff, 44
Biden, Joe, 47, 65, 79, 81, 139–40
bilingualism: of COVID-19 vaccine communications, 153–54; of Facebook messages from health agencies, 140; of Hispanic reporting, 133–35, 141

Black Coalition Against COVID, 93
Black communities: in Baltimore, 97–98; Black press, 99, 118–23; Capital B (nonprofit digital start-up), 6, 122–23, 152; Charleston *Post and Courier* partnerships to focus on, 38; COVID-19 pandemic reporting and, 121–22; COVID-19 vaccine disinformation and, 74, 89, 93; health causes of death in, 2; health reporting in, 123; history of Black papers, 121; underrepresentation in mainstream media, 119–20
Black Lives Matter movement, 119
Bloomberg, Michael, 107
Bluesky, 140
Box Elder News Journal, 30
brandjacking, 25
breaking news, 18–19, 39, 55, 101
Brill, Steven, 72
Broder, David, 48
Brumfiel, Geoff, 1
Buffett, Warren, 12
Burstin, Helen, 92

cable TV news, 45, 47–48
Cafecito Nevada (radio show/podcast), 135
California, 26, 34
Cambridge Social Decision-Making Lab, 86
Campante, Filipe, 45
cancer treatment, 2–3, 71
Capital B (nonprofit digital start-up), 6, 122–23, 152
Capitolist (news site), 24
Carlson, Tucker, 49
Caulfield, Mike, 161
CBS Evening News, 47
Center for Countering Digital Hate, 73
Centers for Disease Control and Prevention (CDC), 2, 152; CDC Foundation, 145; *Morbidity and Mortality Weekly Report*, 55–56
Charles, J. Brian, 107–8
Charleston Gazette-Mail (West Virginia), 9–11, 17, 104
Chen, Angela, 21–22
Chen, Caroline, 101
Cheney, Liz, 91

Chequeado (Argentina-based), 82
Chicago Tribune, 15–17
Children's Health Defense, 32
Chilton family's ownership of *Charleston Gazette-Mail*, 9–10
China: COVID-19 and, 17, 24, 42, 80, 82; disinformation from, 23, 74
Chokshi, Dave, 89
City Bureau (Chicago newsroom), 111
City University of New York, 121–22, 133
ClearHealthCosts, 113–14
climate change: Charleston's *Post and Courier* coverage of local health impact, 39; fact checking and, 79, 82; fake news and, 25, 48; false equivalence and, 30–31; farming and, 110–11; SciLine on, 159
clinicians. *See* medical professionals, playbook for
Clinton, Bill, 20
Clinton, Hillary, 46–47, 82
CNN, 64
Coalition for Trust in Health and Science, 160
Coalition in Health and Science, 89–90
collaborations. *See* partnerships and collaborations
Columbia Journalism Review, 28–29, 125
Columbia Journalism School's Tow Center for Digital Journalism, 23
common sense, 160–61
Commonwealth Fund survey on public misunderstanding of ACA, 29
community journalism, 117–36
community partnering with health agencies, 140
conservative news and talk shows: "slime" sites, 23–25; talk radio, 18–20, 45–46; TV broadcasting, 21; on 2022 elections, 24; websites, 23. *See also* Fox News
conspiracy theories: anti-vaxxers and, 68–69, 73; disinformation and, 87
Contacto con Luz (Las Vegas radio show), 132
Contraception (journal), 30
Coppins, McKay, 16
Cornell University, 22
#CoronaVirusFacts alliance, 82

Council of Medical Specialty Societies, 91–92
COVID-19 pandemic: Atlas as Fox News medical expert on, 75; Black Coalition Against COVID, 93; China and, 17, 24; ClearHealthCosts coverage of, 113–14; communicating with public as first therapeutic intervention, 138; #CoronaVirusFacts alliance, 82; deaths from, 1–2, 8, 102; drug abusers' harm reduction measures, 82; Facebook warnings of risks, 84–85; fact checking during, 79–80; failure of communication at start of crisis, 5; false equivalence, consequences of, 31–32; farm workers and food industry workers and, 110; fear, resentment, and anger over, 50; Fox News' coverage of, 49–50; global spread of misinformation, 83; health agencies partnering with community leaders to spread message, 140; health care reporting boosted by, 49, 55; health workers' deaths, reporting on, 102; Hispanic communities and, 135; home care workers and, 129; ivermectin disinformation, 13–14, 31–32, 34–35, 55; local fake news on, 24; major national broadcast outlets disseminating misinformation and disinformation, 48; masks and public health measures, 65–66, 138; media credibility and, 66; mental health and, 129; misinformation's consequences, 8, 138; Native American communities and, 118, 123–25; patient-doctor relationship and acceptance of information, 85, 150–51; politicizing effect of, 42, 49–50, 53, 55–56, 76; pregnancy and, 129; in prisons, 106–7; public health guidance, changes in, 53; racial inequities of, 119, 121–22; radio news on, 19; 2020 election and, 47
COVID-19 vaccines: Black community and, 74, 89, 93; Bloomberg School of Public Health campaign "How to Talk to Friends and Family About COVID-19 Vaccines," 148–49; Carlson's advocacy against, 49; Dover (nurse) receiving during rollout, 7, 67–70, 76; engendering opposition to routine childhood vaccines, 88; Facebook on acceptance rates, 85; fact checking, 80; Illinois Medical Professionals Action Collaborative Team's debunking materials and vaccine information, 153–54; improved rates, effective measures for, 144–45, 153; minority communities and, 74, 135; misinformation about, 1, 3, 7, 49, 67–70, 89, 94–95, 135; nursing homes and, 2; pregnancy and, 129; public health officials, harassment and threats against, 34–35; This Is Our Shot (national campaign), 145; vilification of those reporting on, 66; "wait and see" population and, 77. See also anti-vaxxers
Cranky Uncle (online game), 158
CRAP Test to evaluate websites, 161
credible sources, strengthening of, 23, 78, 90–93
criminal justice, 105–7
critical thinking, 159
crowdsourcing, 83, 94, 113–14
Cuban Americans, 133
Cut, The (women-oriented publication), 127
cynicism. *See* negativity and cynicism

Dallas Morning News, 34
Daniels, Serena Maria, 131
de Beaumont Foundation, 145
debunking, 78, 80–81, 84–86; academic institutions' role in, 146; backfire effect, 85, 144, 151; ephemeral effect, 85; Illinois Medical Professionals Action Collaborative Team and, 153; Public Good Projects and, 90; repetition of, 85, 151. *See also* prebunking
deepfakes, 72, 84
democracy's requirement for truth, 71
democratization of information, 4
Democrats: Affordable Care Act and, 28; attacks on the press, 63; inability to agree with Republicans on facts, 4; Medicaid and, 34; presidential primary race (2008), 46

demonization of the media, 63–66
Detroit and coverage of Hispanic communities, 131
Digiday on diversity in newsroom, 122
DiResta, Renée, 4, 70, 138
disinformation: consequences of, 31, 70; dearth of good local reporting and, 14; defined, 73; distinguished from misinformation, 73, 158; equity and, 74–75; goals of, 70; health agency's strategy to counter, 143; key tools of, 87; major national broadcast outlets disseminating, 48; podcasts and, 61; rationality and objectivity as irrelevant, 86; reporting on, 7, 67; tools to counter, 7, 77–93, 143–45. *See also* fake news; *specific tools to counter*
Disinformation Governance Board (proposed), 93
Dobbs v. Jackson Women's Health Organization (2022), 112, 123, 127–28
Documenters, 111–12
Dover, Tiffany, 7, 67–70, 76, 154
Downie, Leonard, Jr., 13
DROG (Dutch media collective), 86
drug overdose, 2, 58, 97, 99
Duke-Margolis Health Policy Center, 139–40
Duke Sanford School of Public Policy: DeWitt Wallace Center for Media and Democracy, 23; Duke Reporters' Lab, 83–84
Dunn, Tim, 23

Ebola, 31, 101, 118
El Misisipí (Spanish-language newspaper), 130
El Nuevo Herald (Miami), 131, 133
email chain letters, 81
emotional reactions, 50, 86, 160
environmental pollution as public health issue, 110
equity issues, 74–75, 126, 128–30
errors: correction of, 141–43; in health reporting, 26–29; misinformation as, 72–73
ethnic communities. *See* racial and ethnic populations

European Union's Digital Services Act (2023), 94
Everytown for Gun Safety, 107
evidence-based messages, 29, 85, 139, 147, 154
extreme risk protection orders, 59–60
Eyre, Eric, 6–7, 9–11, 14, 39, 104, 184n21

Facebook (now Meta), 3, 5, 10; advertising revenue lost by newspapers to, 37; Brand Lift Survey tool, 149; campaign ads on, 25; COVID-19 information on, 84–85, 149; debunking on, 85; fact checking and, 80; health agency's presence on, 140; misinformation on, 150; as source of health news, 66
fact checking, 78–84, 86, 88, 94, 142, 144, 157–58
FactCheck.org, 3, 81–82, 157
Factchequeado, 82–83, 88, 157
Fairness Doctrine, 45–46
fake news: *Bad News* (game) and, 86; criminal activity of fake sites, 25; fact checking and, 81; from foreign adversaries, 23; longevity of and engagement with, 71–72; money-making from, 25; podcasts and, 61; Trump and, 25, 64–65. *See also* disinformation
false equivalence, 13, 29–32
Fauci, Anthony, 65, 80, 82
fear, 50, 86, 160
Federal Communications Commission, 19–20, 45, 154
First Draft News, 74, 87
Fitzsimon, Chris, 111–12
Floodlight (environmental news cooperative), 25
Florida Power and Light, 24–25
Floyd, George, murder of, 106, 119
Food and Drug Administration, 1, 41
Food & Environment Reporting Network (FERN), 6, 109–11
Fox 8 Live (New Orleans), 114
Fox News, 45–50, 64, 75
Freedom of Information Act requests, 110
freedom of speech issues, 93–94, 155

Freedom's Journal (first US Black newspaper), 121
free or affordable access to good information, 99, 103, 112, 156–57. *See also* paywalls
Fromartz, Sam, 109–11
Frontline: COVID-19 Critical Care Alliance, 13–14; Marshall Project partnership, 105
Furfaro, Hannah, 36–37

Gallup polls on trust: in American institutions, 4; in local news reporting, 11; in the media, 65; in medical system, 3
games online as inoculation against misinformation, 86–87, 158
gender inequities, 128–30. *See also* LGBTQ+ communities; 19th, the; women
ghost papers, 12
global warming. *See* climate change
Gloninger, Chris, 31
Goldstein, Amy, 56–57
Google, 37, 80, 84, 91
Gorka, Sebastian, 20
Gorman, Sara, 4–5, 74
Gounder, Celine, 59–60
Go Viral! (online game), 86–87, 158
Graham, Garth, 92
Graham, Lindsey, 155
Gray, Luz, 132–36
Ground Truth Project, 35
Guardian, The, partnership with KFF Health News, 102
gun violence, 26, 59–60, 107–9, 112, 141, 149–50
Gusman (graphic design agency), 86

harassment and threats: against medical clinicians on social media, 151; against public health officials, 34–35, 49, 65, 80, 144
Harmony Square (online game), 87, 158
Harvard Public Health Magazine, 110
Harvard T. H. Chan School of Public Health, 139–40
hate speech, 94
health agencies, playbook for, 138–46; avoiding reporters, 142–43; backfire effect of debunking, 144; closed information groups, dissemination to, 141; communications office, need for, 145–46; community collaboration, 140; context for news and background briefing, 139; correction of misinformation and errors, 141–43; distortion and misinformation, strategy to counter, 143–45; elements of effective communications strategy, 139–40, 145; fact checking, 144; harassment and threats, need to respond to, 144; network development to share messages, 144–46; ongoing creation of content, 145; prebunking, 143–44; social media, use of, 140; speed of response, 143, 145
health consequences of collapse of local news, 13, 25–35, 38; less accountability, 33–35; less awareness, 25–26; more distrust, 32–33; more errors in reporting, 26–29; more false equivalence, 29–32
Hemmer, Nicole, 55
Heritage Foundation, 45–46
Hill-Harris survey on public views of news media, 64–65
Hispanic American communities: Charleston *Post and Courier* partnerships to focus on, 38; diabetes as cause of death, 2; disinformation and, 74, 135; fact-checking sites for, 82–83, 157; news media giving voice to, 118, 120, 130–35; nonprofit news in, 99, 131
HIV, 31, 88, 106, 122
Hojman, Daniel, 45
homeland security, 93
Hoover Institution, 75
Hot Farm (podcast), 110–11
Hunt, Dianna, 8, 117–18, 124–26, 136
Hurricane Harvey (2017), 118

ICT (formerly *Indian Country Today*), 8, 117–18, 123–26; Cronkite School of Journalism and Mass Communication partnership, 126; physicians reprinting articles for patients, 152; reaching wider audiences, 126, 136
Idaho, 28, 34–35

ideologically driven networks, 5, 137
iHeard St. Louis, 89
Illinois Medical Professionals Action Collaborative Team, 153–54
immigrants and immigration, 79, 83, 89, 93, 98, 110, 133–34
incrementalist journalism, 58
Indian Country Today. *See* ICT
Indian Health Service, 124–25
Indigenous Journalists Association, 117
IndiJ Public Media, 118
indoor air pollution, 55
infant health and mortality, 2–3, 15
infertility, 39, 74, 88
infodemic, 69–72, 77, 137
information environmentalist, need for, 155
information sickness, 4, 8; as consequence of journalism's decline, 5; people at risk for, 156; preventing in marginalized communities, 136; protection from, 155
innovators, 96–116. *See also* nonprofit media sector
inoculation against misinformation, 86–88, 158. *See also* prebunking
Inside Climate News (nonprofit), 99
Inside Story (video series), 105–6
Instagram, 80, 140, 151
Institute for Nonprofit News, 99, 104–5, 115, 120, 126, 131
International Fact-Checking Network, 82, 157
International Women's Media Foundation, 113
investigative reporting, 100–101
Iran, disinformation from, 23, 74
Isakson, Johnny, 90–91
ivermectin, 13–14, 31–32, 34–35, 55

James, Bronny, 94–95
Jankowicz, Nina, 93
Jezebel (women's publication), 127
Johns Hopkins Medicine guide to symptoms and diseases, 161
Johns Hopkins University, 15, 139–40; Bloomberg American Health Initiative, 97; Bloomberg School of Public Health, 91, 148–50; Center for Gun Violence Solutions, 149–50; Center for Health Security, 77; ICT data on COVID-19 pandemic impact on Native Americans and, 125
Johnson, Ron, 80
Johnston, Abby, 127–28

Kaiser, Cameron, 34
Kaiser Family Foundation. *See* KFF
Kendall, Peter, 16–17
Kennedy, Robert F., Jr., 32, 73
Kerner Commission, 119–20
KESQ News Channel 3 (California), 21
KFF (formerly Kaiser Family Foundation): COVID-19 Vaccine Monitor, 76–77; disinformation initiative, 90; *Health Misinformation Monitor*, 146; KFF Health News, 6, 60, 99, 101–5, 128
King/Drew Medical Center (Los Angeles), 100
Kirk, Charlie, 20
Knight Foundation: philanthropy to local news sector, 115; surveys on trust in local news reporting, 11, 29
Kreuter, Matthew, 89

Lancet study linking vaccination and autism, 31
Lang, Robert, 18–20
Las Vegas and *Nevada Independent en Español*, 132
Latino communities. *See* Hispanic American communities
Leguen, Fermin, 135
Lenfest Institute, 115
LGBTQ+ communities, news media giving voice to, 99, 106, 118, 126–27. *See also* 19th, the; transgender people
liberal news and talk shows: MSNBC, 45; online sites, 23; radio broadcasting, 20, 45
life expectancy inequities, 2–3, 123
Limbaugh, Rush, 20
LinkedIn, 140
Linvill, Darren, 72
local news, collapse of, 5, 7, 9–40, 137; big-city newspapers' influence and, 14–18; consequences of, 12–13, 24;

consolidation of local radio and TV, 18–22; digital circulation, 17; elimination of print editions, 17, 137; "Era of Evil Owners," 17; experienced reporters leaving the field, 22, 27; fact checking and, 83–84; filling the void, 23–25, 111–12; health consequences of, 13, 25–35; initiatives to save local news, 35–40, 115, 154, 161; national news reported instead of local stories, 18, 22; news deserts resulting from, 11–14
Los Angeles Times, 41, 44, 100
Luthra, Shefali, 128–29, 136

MacArthur Foundation, 35
Made to Save coalition, 93
Magee, Fairriona, 108–9
Maldita.es, 82
marginalized communities, news outlets serving, 11, 74–75, 99, 117–36, 139; Black news media, 121–23; Capital B, 6, 122–23, 152; data gaps, 125; diversity in the newsroom, 119–20; fighting misinformation, 119; health agencies seeking exposure in, 75, 141; Hispanic news media, 130–35; impact of reporting, 136; Native American news media, 117–18, 123–26; the 19th (gender inequities), 6, 126–30, 136; restoring trust in media, 119. *See also specific communities*
Margolis, Michele, 51
Marshall Project, 6, 105–7; *Inside Story* (video series), 105–6; *News Inside* (print publication), 105
Massara, Graph, 80–81
Mayo Clinic Health Library (online), 160–61
McDaniels, Andrea, 16, 96–98
McGuire, Tim, 13
measles, 3, 82, 141
Media Impact Funders, 104, 115
mediaQuant on Trump free publicity (2016), 47
MediaWise, 159
Medicaid, 29, 34, 43, 50, 59, 112, 135
medical debt, reporting on, 102
medical procedures, pricing of, 113–14

medical professionals, playbook for, 150–54; avoiding reporters, 154; behavioral theories to improve communication, 152–53; collaboration, 153–54; patients' trust of, 95, 101, 150–51; reprinting specialty news sites' articles for patients, 152; social media, use of, 151
Medicare, 2, 43, 90, 113
Memes, Magnets and Microchips (Stanford Internet Observatory's Virality Project), 73–74, 88
Memphis Free Speech (Black newspaper), 121
mental health, 3, 26, 36–37, 89, 123, 128–29
Meta. *See* Facebook
Miami Herald, 15, 24; *El Nuevo Herald*, 131, 133
Michigan, COVID-19 policies, 34
misinformation, 67–95; academic challenges, 75, 147; consequences of, 70, 123; on COVID-19 vaccine, 1, 3, 7, 49, 67–70, 89, 94–95, 135; dearth of good local reporting and, 13–14, 22; defined, 72–74, 94; differential susceptibility, 75–77; distinguished from disinformation, 73; evidence-based messages to counter, 147; false equivalence, consequences of, 31–32; global and national agencies countering, 77; government as source of, 71; health agencies countering, 77, 143, 145; infodemic, 69–72, 77, 137; inoculation against, 86–88; longevity of and engagement with, 71–72; major national broadcast outlets disseminating, 48; medical practitioner's credibility countering, 150–51; mobilizing to fight, 78, 93; persuadable population as audience for credible messages, 77; podcasts and, 61; reading the news as way to protect against, 156–57; regulation of, 94–95; self-policing of social media, 94; social media spreading, 5, 31, 71–72, 151; "stickiness" of, 76; targeting minority communities, 7, 119, 123, 135; tools to counter, 7, 77–93, 143–45. *See also specific tools to counter*

Mississippi Today (nonprofit), 99
Monet, Jenni, 124–25
monitoring. *See* surveillance and monitoring
Moonves, Leslie, 47
Morrisey, Patrick, 10–11
Mountain Spotlight, 104, 184n21
Moynihan, Daniel Patrick, 8
MSNBC, 45, 49–50
Murthy, Vivek, 53
Musk, Elon, 94–95

National Academy of Medicine (NAM), 91–92
National Bureau of Economic Research: on TV cable news' influence on COVID-19 protections, 49–50; working paper (2022), 17–18
National Institute for Health Care Management, 126
National Magazine Award to *News Inside*, 106
National Medical Association, 93
national news, 41–66; "bigfooting" of politics reporters, 56–57; cultural bias, 57–59; demonization of, 63–66; expert journalists' struggles, 59–60; "gotcha" stories, 52–55, 63; "Outrage Machine" and, 50; polarized networks, 48–50, 137; policy coverage's demotion, 55–57, 137; polls, effect of, 51–52; rise of talk shows and polarization in, 44–48; shrinkage and buyouts of, 44, 56, 97, 154; verticals, limitations of, 60–63; wire services and, 41–42
National Public Radio (NPR), 1, 25, 55, 61, 103
National Trust for Local News, 35
Native Americans: COVID-19 pandemic and, 118, 123–24; data gaps, 125; health issues of, 124; Hunt as Native American journalist, 117–18; life expectancy of, 2, 123; news outlets giving voice to, 120, 123–26; nonprofit news sector and, 99; as survivors of genocide, forced relocation, and cultural suppression, 123; underrepresentation in mainstream media, 124

negativity and cynicism, 7, 28, 46, 51, 54–55, 58, 63, 81, 158, 160
Nevada, Hispanic and rural reporting in, 132–35
Nevada Independent, 132
Nevada Independent en Español, 6, 132–35, 141
New England Journal of Medicine, 92
New Orleans Tribune (Black newspaper), 121
New Republic, 110
news avoidance, 6, 58
news deserts, 11–12, 35, 38, 83, 116, 161
NewsGuard, 72, 159
News Inside, 105
news literacy, development of, 159–60
News Literacy Project, 159
NewsMatch, 115
New York Amsterdam News (Black newspaper), 121
New York City's Department of Health and Mental Hygiene, Community Concerns Team, 89
New York Public Radio, 114
New York Times: "Dying Broke" series (with KFF Health News), 102; health reporting by, 55; investigative journalism fellowship to bolster local news, 98–99; Marshall Project partnership, 105; on Medicaid plans, 34; opioid reporting, collaboration with *Baltimore Banner*, 7, 115; underrepresentation of minority journalists at, 120; Upshot, 61–62; *Well* (newsletter), 62
19th, the (women and LGBTQ+'s national news organization), 6, 126–30; abortion access and, 127–28; asterisk in name, 127; impact of reporting, 136; as parachute-free zone, 129–30; trans community's access to health care, 130
Nixon, Richard, 63
NOLA.com, 114
nonprofit media sector, 6, 35–40, 96–116, 138–39; challenges ahead, 114–16; ClearHealthCosts, 113–14; diversity in the newsroom, 120; Documenters, 111; Food and Environment Reporting Network, 6, 109–11; free access, 99, 103; Marshall Project, 6, 105–7; partnerships

with larger news outlets, 102–4, 114–15; philanthropy to support, 12, 36–37, 98, 102, 104–5, 113, 115; ProPublica and KFF Health News, 6, 34, 60, 99–105, 115; Report for America, 35, 115; significance of, 116; single-subject focus of, 104; States Newsroom, 111–12; subscription to, 161; Trace, 6, 107–9, 122, 141. *See also Baltimore Banner*
NORC at the University of Chicago, 115
Northwestern University, 12

Obamacare. *See* Affordable Care Act
Offit, Paul, 31–32
Ofori-Atta, Akoto, 122–23
Oklahoma's abortion ban, 128
online games as inoculation against misinformation, 86–87, 158
opioids: addiction and role of drug distributors, 3, 7, 10, 99, 184n21; litigation proceeds, 33
Ornstein, Charles, 100–101
Orthodox Jewish communities, 89, 141
outliers as good stories, 60

parachuting coverage of hot stories, 129
partnerships and collaborations: Food & Environment Reporting Network (FERN) and, 110; health agencies and, 144–45; ICT and, 126; KFF model of, 102–4; Marshall Project and, 105, 107; nonprofits and, 102–4, 114–15
patient-doctor relationship, 76, 85, 150–52
Patterson, Thomas, 54–55
paywalls, 63, 123; access without, 62, 99, 112, 135
PBS, 44
Pew Charitable Trust's Stateline (online news), 112
Pew surveys: health policy in 2016 presidential election, 46; on Hispanic media, 131; on job loss of local reporters, 12; on radio listening audience, 18; on Republicans and Democrats unable to agree on facts, 4
Philadelphia Center for Gun Violence Reporting, 26

philanthropies. *See* nonprofit media sector
physicians. *See* medical professionals, playbook for
Pinder, Jeanne, 113–14
"pink slime," 23–25
Pittsburgh Courier (Black newspaper), 121
playbook for health communication, 137–55; for academic institutions, 146–50; for clinicians and health care organizations, 150–54; for health agencies, 138–46; for policymakers, 154–55
podcasts, 61, 85
polarization, 44–50, 87
policymakers, playbook for, 154–55
politicized content: health care reporting and, 42; horse-race stories, 44, 47, 51, 57, 142; polarization, increase in, 45; radio broadcasting, 20; 2022 elections, biased pseudo-sites delivering, 24
Politico, 55–56, 59, 62–63
PolitiFact, 81–83, 157
Post and Courier (Charleston, SC), 115; investigative reporting initiative, 37–40; "Rising Waters" initiative, 39; "Uncovered" project, 38–40
Poynter Institute, 82, 157, 159. *See also* PolitiFact
prebunking, 78, 86–88, 90, 143–44, 158
presidential elections: perpetual campaigning, 47; 2016, 46–47, 50; 2020, 47. *See also* politicized content
Press Forward, 35
press releases and press conferences, 138–39, 145
prisons and prisoners, 105–7
ProPublica, 6, 34, 99–105, 115
protection of news sources, 155
Public Good Project, 90, 145
public health: averting and preventing problems, 59; COVID-19 pandemic politicizing, 42, 49–50, 53, 55–56, 76; FERN and, 110; officials and experts, harassment and threats against, 34–35, 49, 65, 80, 144; SciLine on, 159; workforce shortage, 49. *See also* health agencies, playbook for

Pulitzer Prize winners: Eyre, 6–7, 10–11, 39; Marshall Project, 105; *News Inside*, 106; nonprofit news, 99; Zhu, 99

racial and ethnic populations: COVID-19 pandemic inequities and, 119, 121–22; COVID-19 vaccine disinformation and, 74, 89, 93; "creeping segregation," 98; ethnic media, 120; infant mortality, 15; life expectancy, 2, 123; maternal mortality, 123; racial bias in medicine, 123; systemic racism in criminal justice system, 105–6. *See also* marginalized communities, news outlets serving; *specific races and ethnicities*
radio coverage of local news, 18–20, 45
Ralston, Jon, 132
rapid response. *See* surveillance and monitoring
Reagan, Ronald, 19, 45, 63–64
repetition: of content from academic institution, 148; of debunking, 85, 151; of erroneous or fake news, 29
Report for America, 35, 115
reproductive health, 39, 74, 88, 123, 127. *See also* abortion access
Republicans: Affordable Care Act and, 28, 42, 90–91, 182n76; inability to agree with Democrats on facts, 4; Medicaid and, 34; on news media as the enemy and untrustworthy, 63, 65; opposition to Disinformation Governance Board proposal, 93
Reuters, 157
Rieger, Wendy, 20
Rizzo, Meredith, 1
Robert Wood Johnson Foundation, 58, 76
Roe v. Wade overturned. *See Dobbs v. Jackson Women's Health Organization*
Rogan, Joe, 61
Roozenbeek, Jon, 87
Rosen, Jay, 44, 58
Rosenfeld, Sophia, 71
Rousseau, David, 103–4
rural America, 2, 12, 99, 110, 112, 126, 133
Rural News Network, 126
Russia, disinformation from, 4, 23, 74

Salem Radio Network, 20
Salmon, Daniel, 152–53
Salton Sea, reporting on, 21
Sanders, Bernie, 47
Sanger-Katz, Margot, 61–62
SARS, 31
Schudson, Michael, 13
Schwartzapfel, Beth, 105–7
SciCheck (FactCheck.org), 157
science: attack on credibility of, 2, 70; politicization of, 52–53; public education offerings on, 159
Science on retweeted false stories, 69–70
ScienceUpFirst, 159–60
SciLine, 159
Seattle Times, 36–37, 115
sensationalism, 22, 27, 52
Shorenstein Center on Media, Politics and Public Policy, 47
SIFT model to evaluate websites, 161
Sinclair Broadcast Group, 15, 21
Sinema, Kyrsten, 25
Smith, David, 15, 21
Smith, Keith and Darla, 13–14, 31
smoking. *See* tobacco use
Snipe, Margo, 123
social media: ability to quickly spread misinformation, 5, 31; congressional initiatives to regulate, 155; death of local newspapers and, 11; errors on, 7, 29; expertise in using, 6; fact checking and, 80; harassment and bullying of medical professionals on, 151; health agency's monitoring of, 143; health agency's presence on, 140; health information on, 5, 71; independent regulator proposed for, 155; influencers on, 85; medical professionals fighting misinformation on, 151; profit from disinformation, 70; self-policing of, 94; tags to indicate fact checking, 80. *See also specific platforms*
Solutions Journalism, 58
Soon-Shiong, Patrick, 41
Source NM (New Mexico), 112
South Carolina, accountability and corruption of public officials in, 37–39

Southern Nevada Health District, 135
Southwell, Brian, 69
Spanish-language publications: Anglo-owned, 131, 133; Latino-owned, 131. *See also specific publications by name*
Spectrum (autism publication), 36
Spot the Troll (online game), 158
Stahl, Lesley, 64
Stanford Internet Observatory's Virality Project, 73–74, 88
state government: citizen journalists and, 111; fact checking and, 83–84; Spanish-language reporting on, 134
States Newsroom, 111–12, 184n21
Stirewalt, Chris, 48, 50
Street on Trump's 2016 free ride of media coverage, 47
suicide rates, 2, 26
Sullivan, Margaret, 14
surveillance and monitoring, 78; in health agency's strategy, 143; for rapid response, 89–90, 144–45; real-time monitoring, 145; of social media, 80

talk radio, 18–20, 45–46
Telegram, 88
Telemundo, 131
Tenpenny, Sherri, 31
Texas: Rio Grande Valley's abortion access, 129–30; SB 8 (2021) ban on abortions and civil suits against aiders and abettors, 127–28; trans community's access to health care, 130; underrepresentation of Native reporters, 118
Theranos scandal, 56, 101
Thiel, Peter, 23
This Is Our Shot, 145
TikTok, 80, 87, 140, 150
Times-Picayune, 114
tobacco use, 22, 69, 123
Toff, Benjamin, 6, 58
tools to counter disinformation and misinformation, 7, 77–93, 143–45. *See also* debunking; evidence-based messages; fact checking; prebunking
Tostada Magazine, 131
Trace, The, 6, 107–9, 122, 141

Trahant, Mark, 117
transgender people, 48, 129–30. *See also* 19th, the
transparency, 33, 94, 98, 114–15, 143, 147–48
Tropes & Stereotypes (newsletter), 108
Trump, Donald: ACA attacked by, 28; antagonism toward reporters, 63–66; Atlas as health adviser to, 75; as "Bottomless Pinocchio," 79; COVID-19 reporting and, 55–56, 65–66; fact checking of, 79; fake news and, 25, 64–65; pandemic and, 53–54, 79; polarization of American politics and, 50; on Republican Party, 82; stolen election and January 6 claims of, 91; Twitter and Fox News catering to, 64; 2016 election, 46–47, 50; 2020 election, 48
Trusting News, 159
trust issues: in academic communications, 147–48; in American institutions, 4, 6, 140; Black reporting and, 122; Coalition for Trust in Health and Science, 160; democracy and, 71, 122–23; disinformation fostering, 70; Hispanic reporting and, 133, 135; lack of local news reporting, effect of, 10–14, 32–33; in media reporting, 65, 68, 119; in medical practitioner, 95, 101, 150–51; in medical system, 3, 6, 32–33, 70–71, 76, 140, 160; Native American reporting and, 118; in nonprofit media sector, 115; rebuilding trust, 74, 119, 122, 159; in science, 52–53
Tuckson, Reed, 90
TV news: cable TV, 45, 47–50; conservative news and talk shows, 21; consolidation of local radio and TV, 18–22. *See also* Fox News
Twitter (now X), 34; Community Notes, 94–95; fact checking and, 80; health agency's presence on, 140; retweeted false stories, 69–70, 94–95; Trump's use of, 64
Tyndall Report on 2016 election coverage of health policy, 46

Uihlein, Richard, 23
University of Cambridge, 86–87

University of Maryland's health and medicine programs, 15
University of Minnesota, 22
University of Pennsylvania, 66. *See also* Annenberg Public Policy Center
University of Southern California Center for Health Journalism, 21
University of Washington mental health research and programs, 36
Univision, 131–32

vaccines and vaccinations: false equivalence and, 31; free flu vaccination clinics, 140; meningitis B vaccine, 31; misinformation about, 69; opposition to school-age children requirements, 2, 88, 95; polio vaccine, 2; RSV vaccine, 82, 91. *See also* COVID-19 vaccines
van der Linden, Sander, 87
verticals, limitations of, 60–63
Viral Spiral (FactCheck.org), 157
Vox, 60, 122

Wall Street Journal, 55–56
Ward, Ken, Jr., 9
Warren, Elizabeth, 155
Washington (state), mental health care in, 36–37
Washington Post: Bezos as owner, 44; fact-check feature of, 79–80, 158; health reporting by, 55–57; *Health 202* (online newsletter), 61; on life expectancy decline, 3; Maryland coverage, 97; *Wonkblog*, 61
Washington University in St. Louis's Brown School of Public Health, 89
Washoe County Health District (Nevada), 135
WBAL (Baltimore NewsRadio), 18–20
Wells, Ida B., 121
Wesleyan University, 22
West Virginia Watch, 184n21
WhatsApp, 5, 70, 83, 88, 141, 150
White, Gillian, 122
White House reporters, 56–57, 64–65
Whitmer, Gretchen, 34
Williams, Lauren, 122–23
wire services, 7, 10, 41–42
women: news media giving voice to, 99, 118. *See also* abortion access; 19th, the; reproductive health
World Health Organization (WHO), 70–71, 86–87, 91–92, 158
WyoFile, 112

X (formerly Twitter). *See* Twitter

Young, Dannagal Goldthwaite, 48
YouTube, 66, 87–88, 91–92, 138, 140–41

Zadrozny, Brandy, 7, 67–69, 95
Zhu, Alissa, 7, 96, 98–99, 115–16
Zika, 31
Zommer, Laura, 83

Browse more books from HOPKINS PRESS

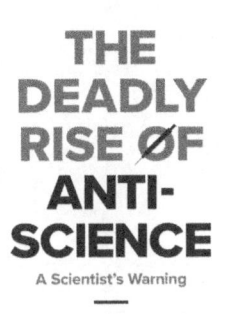

"A powerful eyewitness account of anti-scientific activities in the USA."

—Naomi Oreskes,
The Lancet

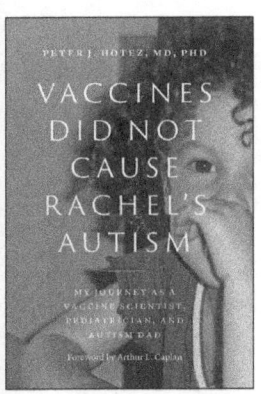

"Hotez isn't pulling any punches."

—*Foreword Reviews*

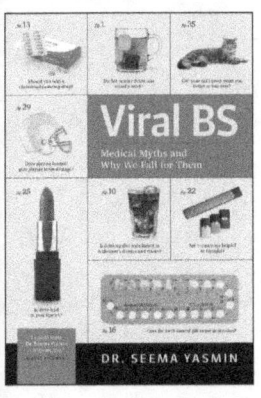

"Brilliant, hilarious, infuriating, and illuminating, Viral BS is essential reading for anyone with a brain and internet access."

—*Melody Moezzi*,
author of *The Rumi Prescription*

JOHNS HOPKINS UNIVERSITY PRESS | PRESS.JHU.EDU